ESSENTIAL KETOGENIC DIET PRESSURE COOKING

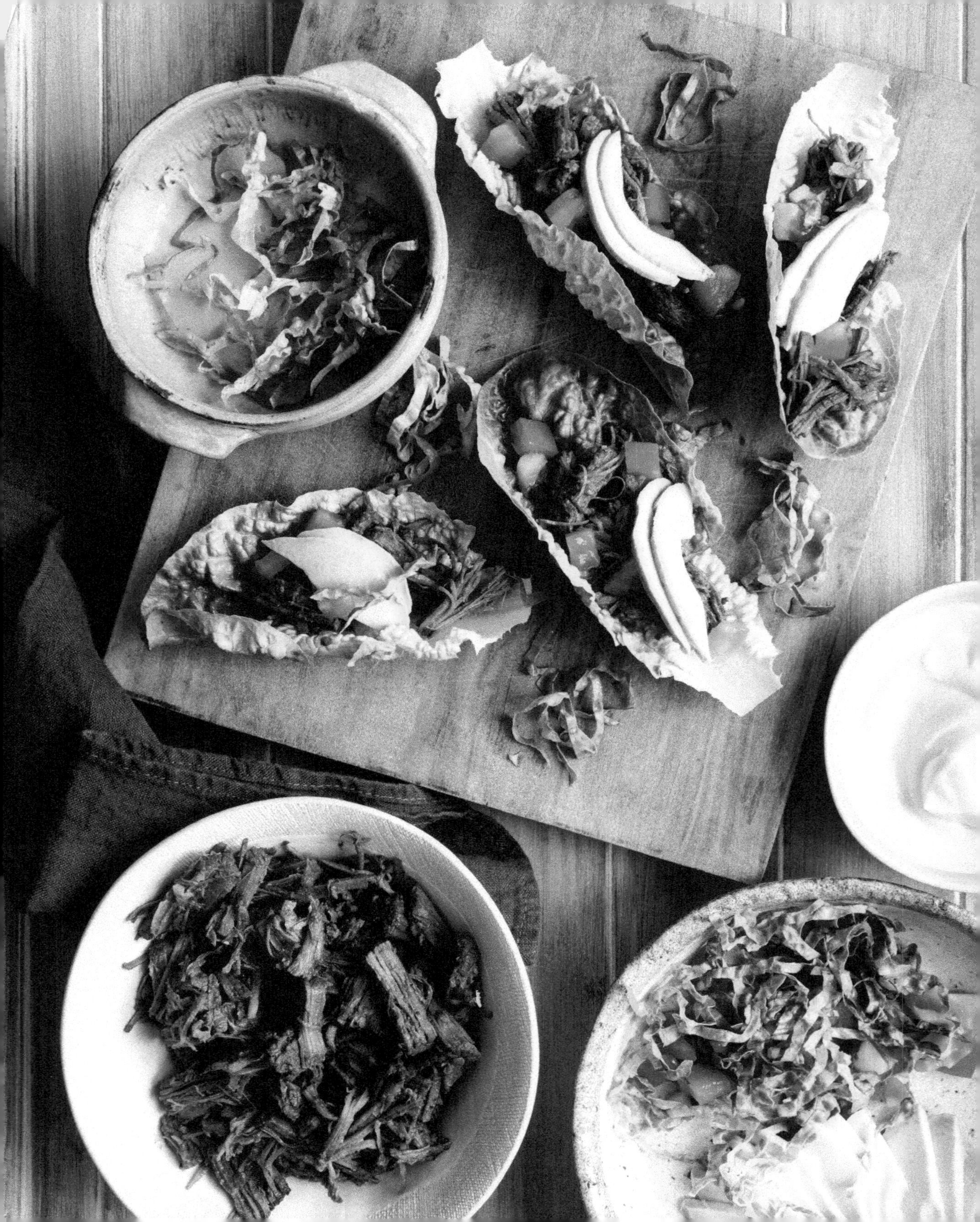

ESSENTIAL Ketogenic Diet PRESSURE COOKING

Low-Effort, Big-Flavor Keto Recipes for Any Pressure Cooker or Multicooker

JANE DOWNES

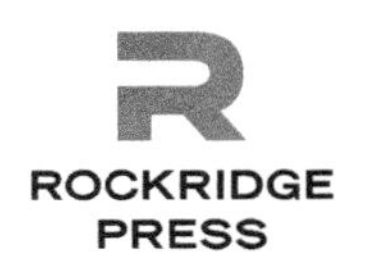

For general information on our other products and services or to obtain technical support, please contact our Customer Care Department within the United States at (866) 744-2665, or outside the United States at (510) 253-0500.

Rockridge Press publishes its books in a variety of electronic and print formats. Some content that appears in print may not be available in electronic books, and vice versa.

Designer: Katy Brown
Editor: Stacy Wagner-Kinnear
Production Editor: Erum Khan

Cover photography © Marija Vidal, 2018; food styling by Cregg Green

Cover: Whole Chicken, page 106 and Bacon Brussels Sprouts, page 56

ISBN: Print 978-1-93975-440-0
eBook 978-1-93975-441-7

For Mom and Dad

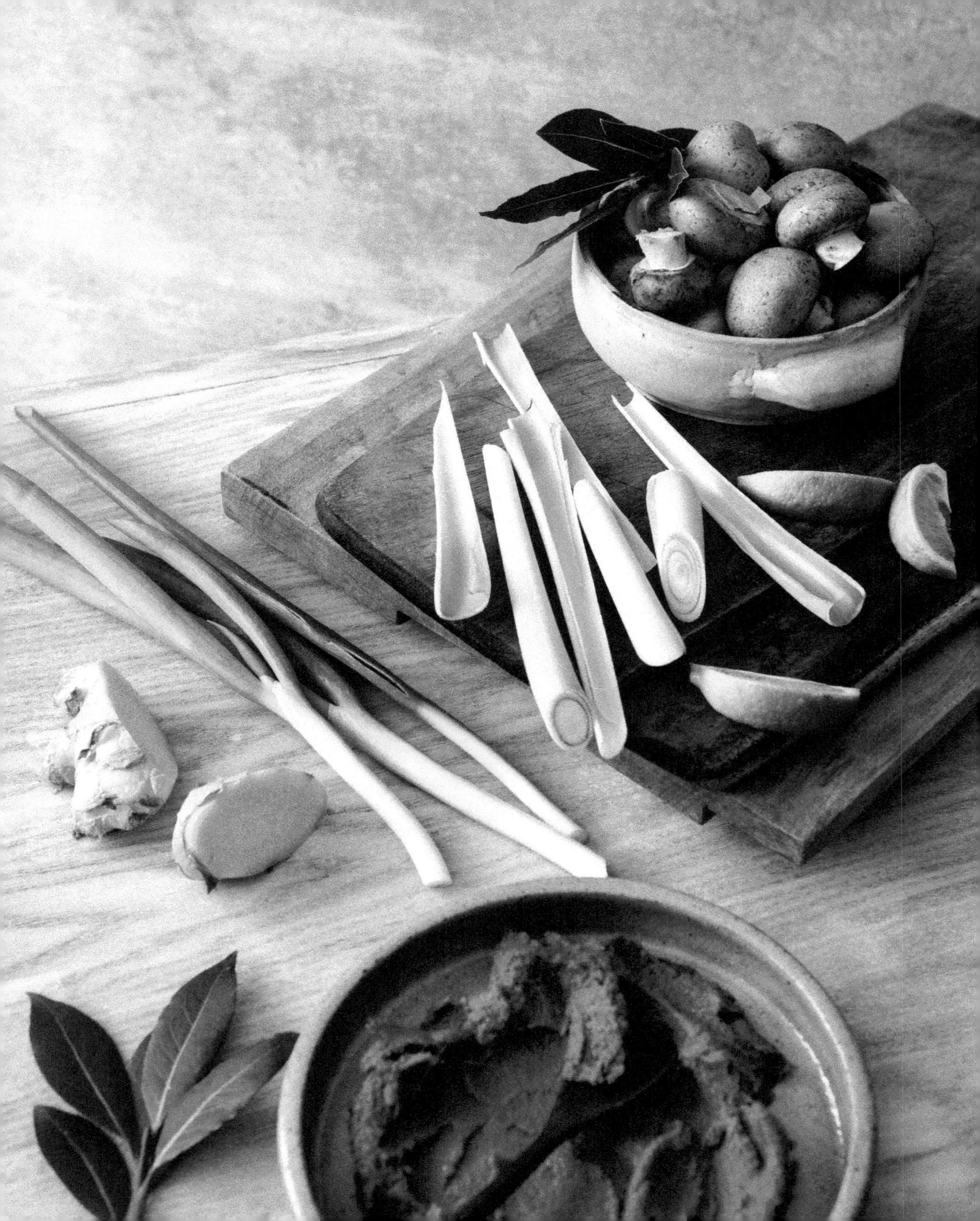

CONTENTS

INTRODUCTION

I have been working as a personal trainer and nutrition coach since 2013, but only discovered the ketogenic diet in late 2015. I was in search of relief from my depression and anxiety through a non-medication approach. I not only saw the results I was looking for but also experienced improved body composition, sustainable energy, improved digestion and skin, and a list of other wonderful health benefits. I then spent the following years learning everything I could about this lifestyle and the possible implications it could have for me and my clients. After diving headfirst into educating myself on all things keto, I started implementing a ketogenic or low-carb lifestyle with the appropriate clients. I continued to discover the power this style of eating has to change someone's health. The majority of my work is now specialized in implementing low-carb and ketogenic nutritional protocols with clients to help them achieve their desired health and overall well-being goals. I do this work through multiple platforms, including in-person one-on-one coaching, remote online coaching, and with FitKetoGirls, a company I co-founded with my business partner and wonderful friend, Liz Williams.

Cooking has always been a passion of mine, and when I started eating a ketogenic diet this passion amplified. Prior to eating a ketogenic diet I ate a more conventional low-fat, high-carbohydrate diet. I also ate five to six meals a day. The restricting breakdown of my macronutrients (carbs, proteins, fats) and the frequency of my meals resulted in me eating bland combinations of plain rice, steamed veggies, and lean proteins. I also often felt restricted and unsatisfied with my food. Making the switch to a high-fat lifestyle with less meal frequency brought back flavor and my love for food. Because with keto I only eat two to three times a day, I now have the time to spend cooking and experimenting with the wonderful world of ketogenic and low-carb cooking. I incorporated fat and salt back into my cooking, which brought back all the flavor to my meals. I enjoyed the food I was eating, and this healed my once unhealthy relationship with food. Cooking and mealtime has become time I truly treasure each day. There are few things I find more rewarding than creating high-fat, nutrient-dense meals and sharing these recipes with my loved ones.

My love for cooking led the way to my more recent love for my Instant Pot® multicooker, which I purchased mainly for its pressure cooking functionality. I'd been using a slow cooker quite a bit, but I always wanted the meat to cook faster. The Instant Pot has quickly become my main cooking appliance. Using a pressure cooker means that my meals can be prepared faster and with more flavor than I'd get with stove top or oven cooking. Because of this new obsession, I have created this cookbook of all of my favorite high-fat recipes for you to enjoy. You can use these recipes with any version of a pressure cooker you own, including the Instant Pot, Power Pressure Cooker XL, or a stove-top pressure cooker. This cookbook will help you learn how to make keto-compliant recipes with confidence.

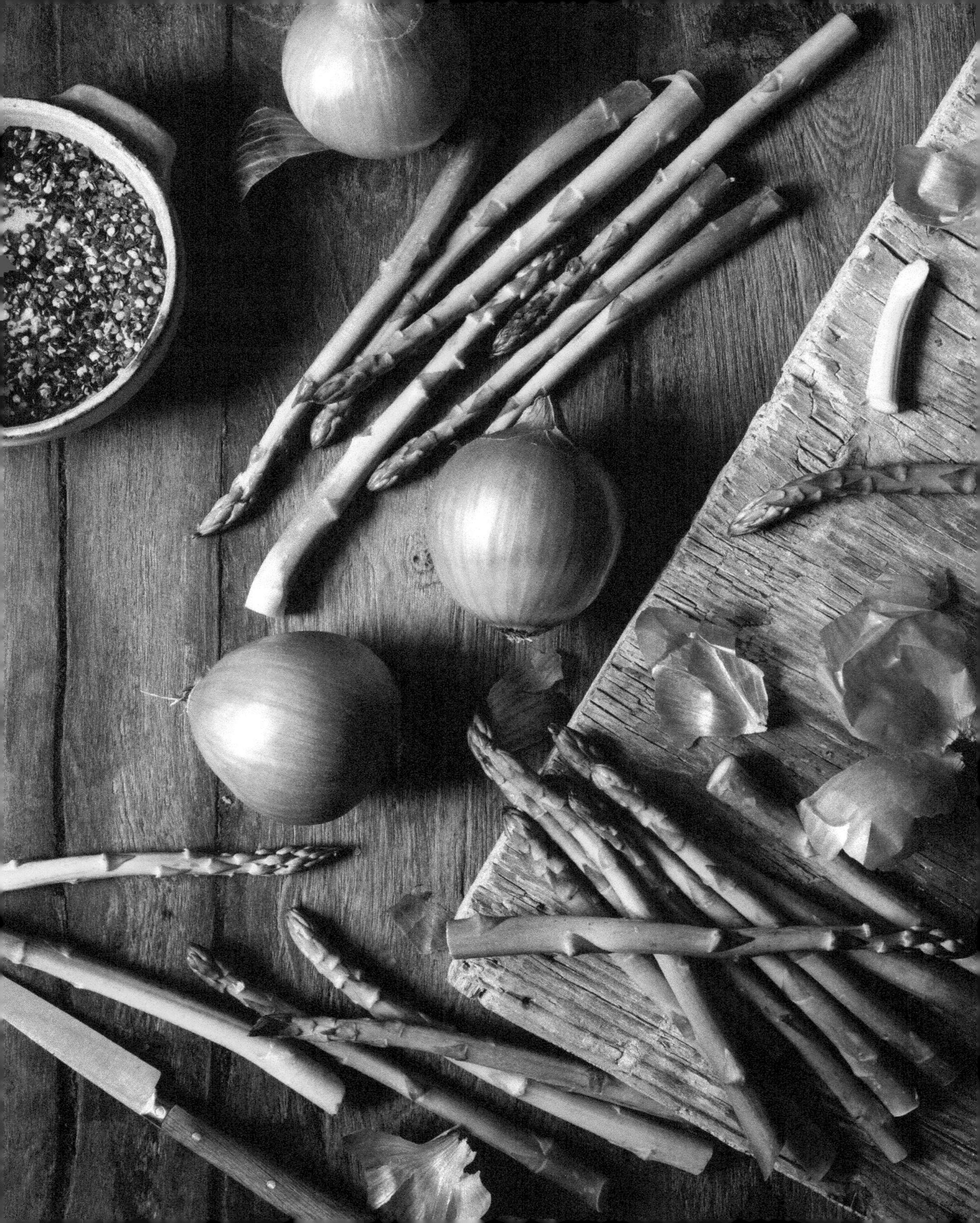

Chapter One

Keto Pressure Cooking 101

DID AN AMAZON PRIME DEAL convince you to purchase the Instant Pot but you're not quite sure how to maximize its use while eating keto? I am here to show you how all of your keto staples and favorites can come together faster and easier than you thought possible.

The ketogenic diet is an amazing lifestyle that I have implemented with hundreds of clients. However, one complaint I hear about the diet is its lack of variation in foods and recipes. Everyone loves bacon and eggs at first, but over time people can experience some food fatigue. This recipe book is here to change that, giving you endless flavors and recipe variations to ensure that you make the best use of your pressure cooker to keep keto interesting and satisfying.

KETO IN BRIEF

I'm guessing this book isn't your introduction to keto, but it's good to establish common principles and understandings right from the start. The ketogenic diet is a high-fat, moderate-protein, low-carb style of eating used to achieve the fat-burning metabolic state of ketosis. To formulate an optimal ketogenic diet, you should eliminate grains, sugars, and refined vegetable oils and eat a diet consisting of quality-sourced meats and fish, nutrient-dense vegetables, and healthy fat sources. The macronutrient breakdown is typically 65 to 75 percent fat, 15 to 30 percent protein, and 5 to 10 percent carbohydrates. Eating in this fashion switches your body's metabolic pathway from primarily sugar burning to primarily fat burning. Instead of breaking down carbohydrates into glucose for fuel, your liver will convert fatty acids into ketone bodies to be used as your body's primary fuel source. This style of eating has been shown to have numerous health benefits. Some of the most common are improved brain function, better body composition, increased energy, and decreased inflammation.

MY NUTRITION PHILOSOPHY

Nutrition is not a one-size-fits-all approach, and we each require an individualized nutrition strategy to match our genetic makeup, activity level, and goals. Nothing is going to work for everyone, and it's important to discover what works best for you and your own body and goals. I work with my clients on a very individualized basis and implement a dietary strategy that will best fit the needs and goals of each client.

I have seen incredible results implementing the keto diet with my clients. I believe wholeheartedly in the power of this style of eating and have learned a few tips along the way to help you find success.

EAT REAL FOOD. Just because it's keto does not mean it is healthy. It is very possible to be in a state of ketosis and not consume a nutrient-dense diet. You could easily follow the same macronutrient profile as described above by eating processed cheese wrapped in processed meat or other unhealthy processed foods with ketogenic macronutrients. Instead of this approach, I am a firm believer in choosing the most nutrient-dense sources of fats, proteins, and carbs to construct your ketogenic diet. This means the majority of your food does not have an ingredient list or come out of a bag or box and is not just keto-fied high-carb recipe remakes (keto pizza, keto ice cream, etc.). Rather, your diet consists of quality meats and fish, fresh and nutrient-dense vegetables, and healthy fat sources.

QUALITY, QUALITY, QUALITY. Choosing the right types of foods is very important, but just as important is the quality of those foods. The way the animals you eat are raised and the produce you eat is grown and processed affects the makeup and nutritional value of those foods. Always choose organic, wild-caught, pasture-raised, locally raised, and grass-fed options.

CHOOSE THE RIGHT FAT. Eating a ketogenic diet results in your body using either dietary fat or body fat for its primary fuel source. The types of fats you eat to formulate your high-fat diet are extremely important. I might sound like a broken record, but that is because of the importance of this topic and how frequently I believe it is overlooked. I can't stress enough the importance of the quality and source of the food you eat. Please eliminate all processed and refined vegetable oils and seed oils from your diet. These types of oils are found in almost all store-bought dressings, condiments, and other processed foods, and are linked to a laundry list of unwanted metabolic and inflammatory conditions. Replace canola oil, corn oil, soybean oil, sunflower oil, and margarine with healthy fats and oils such as avocado oil, coconut oil, olive oil, butter, and ghee.

ENJOY THE JOURNEY. One of my favorites things about this lifestyle is how easy it is to maintain and how delicious and satisfying the meals taste. It truly brought back my love for cooking and helped heal my broken relationship with food from chronic dieting. It is imperative to find a way to enjoy this style of eating and have flexibility within the lifestyle. I never want your food to cause additional stress to your life or for you to have the feeling that you are extremely restricted by the parameters of keto. Always be kind and gentle with yourself. Focus on progress and not perfection, and make the best choice you can in the moment. That choice might be a jelly-filled, powdered sugar–covered doughnut once in a while, and that is totally okay, too. While I am obviously passionate about the first few tips, this one is maybe the most important. Food should never be the enemy; instead it should help you achieve your goals and optimize your health.

WHY PRESSURE COOK?

Pressure cookers are a fantastic kitchen appliance for preparing flavorful and fast high-fat, low-carb meals. Before I had my Instant Pot I was using a slow cooker several times a week. My poor slow cooker has not been touched since the Instant Pot arrived (not to mention my stove and oven, which are not receiving much love either). This is because pressure cookers just do it better for the following reasons:

COOKS FOOD FAST: Everyone knows pressure cookers cook food fast, but how much faster? In many cases, food can be cooked 25 to 30 percent faster when compared with stove top or oven cooking.

EASIER AND BETTER: Pressure cookers also often yield better, more consistent results than traditional cooking methods. You may already know that eggs and the pressure cooker are a perfect pairing. By pressure cooking eggs, you save just a minute or two, but the process is entirely hands-off (you never have to worry about water boiling over), and peeling could not be easier. Many people pressure cook their eggs just for the ease of peeling hard-boiled eggs.

ALL IN ONE: Many recipes can be cooked using no other appliances. The Sauté or Browning function of pressure cookers makes cooking one-pot meals easy and efficient.

ENERGY-EFFICIENT: Because pressure cookers cook faster than traditional cooking methods and use significantly less water for cooking, they are among the greenest of all cooking appliances.

FLAVOR- AND NUTRIENT-SAVING: The longer food is exposed to heat, the more nutrients are released. Because of the reduced cooking time in a pressure cooker, foods retain more nutrients and flavor. In addition to the reduced cooking time, steaming vegetables in a pressure cooker requires less water. This in turn results in fewer minerals and nutrients being dissolved. Along with producing more nutrient-dense food, cooking food under pressure infuses it with more intense flavors.

WHAT TO PRESSURE COOK

Pressure cookers cook food using steam and high heat. As a result, pressure cooking works best for recipes and foods that traditionally take a long time to cook and cook in a wet environment. While the pressure cooker will not be your go-to appliance for roasting or grilling, it does excel in quickly cooking braises, soups, stews, sauces, stocks, hard vegetables, dried beans, grains, and legumes. Given that this is a ketogenic cookbook, you won't find out what the pressure cooker does for beans, grains, and legumes, but everything else is fair game.

KETO AND THE COOKER

Pressure cooking and keto are a wonderful match. The ketogenic diet should be formulated by eating quality-sourced meats and fish and fresh and nutrient-dense vegetables that are topped with fat-filled stews, sauces, and condiments. Your pressure cooker can cook all of the above faster and with more infused flavor than conventional cooking methods.

QUALITY-SOURCED PROTEINS

While too much protein on a keto diet isn't a good thing, eating a moderate amount of protein is important to maintain lean mass, and there's nothing better than a pressure cooker for cutting down protein cooking times and cooking each dish to perfection.

EGGS: Hard-boiled and Soft-boiled Eggs (page 28), delicious frittatas, and Avocado Eggs Benedict (page 42) are all cooked to perfection in a pressure cooker. One of my favorite things to cook is hard-boiled eggs because they are "set it and forget it" and are always effortless to peel!

FISH: While it's quick and easy to cook most fish using conventional methods, a pressure cooker is perfect for those days when you've forgotten to defrost something for dinner, since it can cook frozen fish fillets or shrimp beautifully in minutes. And pressure-braising fattier fish like salmon results in a delectably silky texture you won't get from the broiler.

BEEF, PORK, AND POULTRY: The pressure cooker always yields perfectly juicy and tender meat and poultry that is infused with flavor and cooked in a fraction of the time of conventional cooking methods.

HARD VEGETABLES

Low-carb, nutrient-dense vegetables are cooked in just minutes using the pressure cooker. Each of the vegetables below are incredibly easy to cook in the pressure cooker.

- Broccoli florets are cooked in only 1 to 2 minutes.
- Crispy cabbage is done in just about 3 minutes.
- Cauliflower florets are cooked in 2 to 3 minutes, or turned into cauliflower purée in just about 5 minutes.
- Green beans are cooked to perfection in 2 to 3 minutes.

STOCKS, SAUCES, AND CONDIMENTS

Stocks, sauces, and homemade condiments made from healthy fats are the perfect addition to proteins and vegetables, not only to add immense flavor but also to help you hit your fat macronutrients. The pressure cooker's intense cooking environment brings out the deepest, richest flavors in these foods and helps get them cooked faster. These are some of my favorite keto-friendly stocks, sauces, and condiments that you can make in a pressure cooker.

- Beef or chicken stock
- Bone broth
- Bolognese sauce
- Ghee

COMPARING ELECTRIC PRESSURE COOKERS

These days, Instant Pot has become almost synonymous with pressure cooker. While it's true that the brand introduced numerous cooks to pressure cooking, there are many other brands and models. I've included snapshots of several of the more popular brands of electric pressure cookers, all of which happen to be multicookers—that is, they can also sauté, slow cook, and more. Despite the differences I detail, pressure cookers, at their core, all cook the same way.

INSTANT POT

Instant Pot multicookers come in three sizes: 3-quart, 6-quart, and 8-quart. There are several different models with different features. All but the Lux model have adjustable pressure levels (both low and high pressure), and have a yogurt setting. All models come with several preprogrammed settings and have slow-cook settings as well. The Ultra model can also be used for sous vide cooking. In all models, the inner pot is stainless steel, although a ceramic nonstick pot is available separately.

Pros

- Most models can also be used to make yogurt.
- The company has excellent customer service.
- Many accessories are available.

Con

- The preprogrammed settings are not always accurate, and because different models have different preset times, recipes written for the Instant Pot may not work as written for all models.

POWER PRESSURE COOKER XL

This multicooker comes in three sizes: 6-quart, 8-quart, and 10-quart. All have adjustable pressure levels, slow-cook settings, and pre-programmed settings. The inner pot is nonstick.

Pro

- If you want a larger pressure cooker, this brand is one of very few electric cookers that has a 10-quart model.

Con

- The inner pot's nonstick coating is not very durable.

If You Have a Stove-top Pressure Cooker

Now that electric pressure cookers and multicookers have become so popular, many recipes are developed and written for the electric models. But what if you have a stove-top pressure cooker, such as one of the models from popular brands Fagor or Kuhn Rikon? Will foods cook differently?

It's true that most stove-top cookers reach a higher pressure level than most electric models. Pressure level is measured by a term called PSI—pounds per square inch. Stove-top pressure cookers typically reach levels around 15 psi, where electric cookers reach between 9 to 12 psi. But stove-top pressure cookers also generally take less time to come to pressure—and remember, your food is cooking during this time. So, yes, your food will cook at a higher pressure, but it will also cook for less time before it comes to pressure. In my experience, with recipes that require cooking times longer than 10 minutes or so, stove-top and electric cookers will perform the same. That is, you don't have to adjust the cooking time. With recipes that have very short cooking times (0 to 3 minutes), you may need to add a minute if using a stove-top cooker. But remember that you can always cook your food longer after releasing the pressure, so my best advice is to use the times listed and make any adjustments after releasing the pressure.

BREVILLE FAST SLOW PRO

Breville's multicooker comes in one size only: 6-quart. The inner pot is nonstick ceramic. It also functions as a slow cooker and has several preprogrammed settings for both pressure cooking and slow cooking. The pressure level is adjustable.

Pros

- You can choose the release method at the beginning of the cooking cycle.
- The pressure release button is on the front of the machine, so your hand isn't near the steam when you release pressure.

Con

- The lid is attached to the base with an arm that is not detachable. This can make it harder to store.

NECESSARY ACCESSORIES

Give the pressure cooker (and yourself) the gift of the accessories to bring out its best. Note that prices vary all the time with online sales, so keep an eye out and join one or more online communities of fans, who often alert one another to great deals. Here is a list of the best accessories to have and what they help you do or make.

GLASS LID: The glass lid is perfect for when you are using the many other functions of the pressure cooker besides pressure cooking. When using the Sauté setting, the glass lid will keep your food from splattering outside of the pot. The lid can also be used to store the whole inner pot in the refrigerator when storing leftovers.

EXTRA SEALING RING: Over time the sealing ring will absorb the flavors of different foods. Using separate sealing rings for savory and sweet dishes can prevent your cheesecake from tasting like last night's curry.

CUSTARD JARS/MASON JARS/RAMEKINS: These are perfect for making single-serving desserts or single-serving egg dishes.

STEAMER BASKET: A great accessory for steaming vegetables. The basket will ensure that no vegetables fall through and become mush in the water.

7-INCH SPRINGFORM PAN: This is an extremely popular accessory. The 7-inch pan fits perfectly into the pressure cooker and allows you to make delicious cheesecakes and quiches.

SILICONE CUPS: These are perfect for cooking eggs Benedict. They can be used similarly to the custard cups, mason jars, and ramekins, but their flexible surfaces make removing the cooked food much easier.

MEAL PREPPING WITH PRESSURE

Meal planning and prepping is often essential to being successful on a ketogenic diet. With the pressure cooker, meal prep day is about to get a whole lot easier. The set-and-go functions and fast cooking times will allow you to cook more food in less time, without having to stand over a hot stove all day or worry about burning your dishes.

For example, you can easily prep and make several items in one day that you can then enjoy throughout the week. Here I break down a strategy to make Egg Bites (page 40), Hard-boiled Eggs (page 28), Easy Pesto Spaghetti Squash (page 61), Kale and Sausage Soup (page 70), and Balsamic Chicken Thighs (page 118) in one weekend day to have plenty of meals on hand throughout the following week. Here is how I do it:

1. **START OFF THE DAY BY COOKING THE HARD-BOILED EGGS.** This should take about 15 minutes, including the time it takes for the pot to come to pressure. When all the pressure has been released, remove the eggs to a bowl of ice to stop the cooking.

2. **WHILE THE EGGS ARE COOKING, PREP THE VEGETABLES AND SPICES FOR THE OTHER MEALS.** To do so, chop 3 onions, 10 garlic cloves, 6 tomatoes, 6 cups kale, ½ cup baby spinach, and ¼ cup fresh basil. Gather the remaining dry and canned ingredients for the recipes.

3. **PREPARE THE EGG BITES.** Mix and cook the Egg Bites. This should also take about 15 minutes, including the time it takes for the pot to come to pressure. Remove the Egg Bites and let cool before refrigerating for your easy grab-and-go breakfast for the week.
4. **CUT AND REMOVE THE SEEDS FROM THE SPAGHETTI SQUASH AND COOK THE SQUASH.** Prep the Easy Pesto Spaghetti Squash ingredients while the squash cooks, which should take about 20 minutes.
5. **COOK THE SAUSAGE AND KALE SOUP.** This should take about 25 minutes. When done, transfer to individual serving containers and let cool before refrigerating.
6. **MAKE THE BALSAMIC CHICKEN THIGHS.** This should take about 40 minutes. When done, transfer to individual serving containers and refrigerate.

Use these meals throughout the week to make quick and easy keto-friendly choices when you are in a rush, so meal time doesn't have to be stressful. Mix and match your favorite recipes and prep them all at once as outlined above to allow you several grab-and-go options for the week.

FAQS

Below you will find some common questions about ketogenic dieting as well as general pressure cooker questions.

What should my macronutrients be?

The macronutrient breakdown is typically 65 to 75 percent fat, 15 to 30 percent protein, and 5 to 10 percent carbohydrates. However, how this translates into grams of proteins, carbohydrates, and fat needs to be individualized for your body and your goals. I do recommend counting macronutrients, especially in the beginning, to learn how best to formulate your diet. There are several online macro calculators that can be used as a starting point.

Should I count net carbs or total carbs?

There is not a one-size-fits-all approach, but what I typically recommend is counting net carbs for vegetables but total carbs for everything else. I make this recommendation because not all carbs are created equal, and some, like green vegetables, should be included in your ketogenic lifestyle. However, I discourage the consumption of other low-net-carb processed foods like low-carb tortillas or Atkins bars.

Can I eat too much fat?

Yes, you can definitely eat too much fat, and that is why it is important to follow an individualized macro breakdown. If your goal is fat loss, as it is for the majority of my clients, I would recommend only eating fat until satiety. When following a ketogenic lifestyle, your body's main fuel source will be fat, and this can come from dietary fat or body fat. Your body will burn dietary fat first because it is more readily available. If you are overeating dietary fat, you are giving your body no reason to burn body fat. Eating enough fat is important, but overeating fat will not result in fat loss.

Pressure Cooking at High Altitude

The higher the altitude, the lower the atmospheric pressure. With slight changes in altitude, the difference is negligible, but when you get high enough (above 2,000 feet), it can be significant. While the sealed interior of a pressure cooker helps make up for the lower atmospheric pressure, you'll still have to make some adjustments if you live in the mountains. Most pressure cooker manufacturers recommend increasing cooking times by 5 percent for every 1,000 feet above 2,000 feet. Some also recommend increasing the amount of liquid slightly. Check with the manufacturer of your cooker to see if they have any specific recommendations. The Instant Pot Ultra model can be set to adjust automatically for high altitude, but for most cookers, you'll have to adjust the times yourself.

Do calories matter on a ketogenic diet?

Yes. While there is more to fat loss and body recomposition than calories in versus calories out, calories do still matter. Eating too few or eating too many will prevent you from seeing results. Both the number of calories you eat and the types of foods that make up those calories will factor into you seeing results.

For pressure cooking, when should I do a quick release versus a natural release?

Use a natural pressure release for at least 10 to 15 minutes if it can be done without overcooking the dish. Reserve quick release for dishes that require very short cooking times, such as fish, eggs, and tender vegetables or other foods that easily overcook. (I speed it up even more by placing a cold, wet cloth on the lid opposite the pressure release valve, and topping that with a small sealed bag of ice. This method can also be used during natural release to lessen the time it takes.) Quick release is also useful when a dish cooks in stages—if, for instance, the meat component needs to cook longer than the vegetables, I quick release the pressure at the end of the first cooking time, and sometimes at the end of the second cooking time as well.

Can I substitute one cut of meat for another—pork loin for pork shoulder, for instance, or chicken breasts for chicken thighs?

Different meats have varying amounts of connective tissue and fat, which means that they cook at different rates. Substituting one for another is usually possible—it just requires a shorter or longer cooking time. In those cases, check the pressure cooking time charts at the end of this book, or refer to a recipe that you know gives you a reliable cooking time for the cut you have.

How much liquid do I need when pressure cooking? What kind can I use?

A good rule of thumb is to use at least 1 cup of liquid in any recipe, but that amount can include the liquid that's released by meat or poultry as it cooks, so you don't always have to start out with a full cup. For instance, 3 pounds of chuck will release about 2 cups of liquid as it cooks (partially fat-based and partially water-based). In general, using too much liquid is better than too little, since you can pour off or boil off excess liquid after cooking.

As for what kinds of liquids, there's a misconception that only stock or water counts toward that 1 cup of liquid. Some people seem especially wary of using tomato or dairy products, but I don't pressure cook but that use these frequently. I often use diced tomatoes with their juices or strained tomatoes for some or all of my liquid. And if the recipe warrants it, I use milk or cream with no problems.

THIS BOOK'S RECIPES

This cookbook contains all of my favorite pressure cooker recipes, as well as some of my keto diet staples and basics that don't pressure cook but that I use on a regular basis, or that pair perfectly with other recipes included in this book. Here are a few things included in the recipes:

- All recipes specify prep time, cook time under pressure, pressure release method, and total cook time. The time it takes to come to pressure is calculated in the total time as 10 minutes. Many recipes call for a natural release, and that ranges from 10 to 15 minutes. This is included in the total cook time as well.
- Dietary labels are used to let you know if a recipe is dairy-free, gluten-free, nut-free, or vegetarian. (For recipes designated as gluten-free, you should always check ingredient packaging for gluten-free labeling in order to ensure that foods have been processed in a completely gluten-free facility.)
- All nutrition information is listed, including the grams of protein, carbs (both total and net), and fat, as well as the percentages of macronutrients in each serving. No recipe in this book exceeds 12 grams of net carbs.

- I have included tips along the way to provide additional information on ingredients used, substitution options, or cooking techniques. There is also a reference guide in the back of the book for pressure cooking time charts, as well as a list of my favorite keto-friendly resources and brands.
- All of the recipes in this book were tested in my 6-quart Instant Pot DUO60, but they are not written specifically for any one brand of electric pressure cooker. The instructions will work with any type. They will specify the amount of time a recipe cooks under pressure, whether it cooks at high or low pressure, and the method of pressure release you should use. For electric pressure cookers, you'll need to know which setting allows you to manually input the cooking time and pressure level. For stove-top cookers, you'll begin timing after the pressure cooker comes to pressure. In recipes that call for browning foods or reducing sauces, you'll generally use a specific setting on an electric cooker (such as Sauté or Browning), and just heat up the stove-top cooker over medium-high heat.

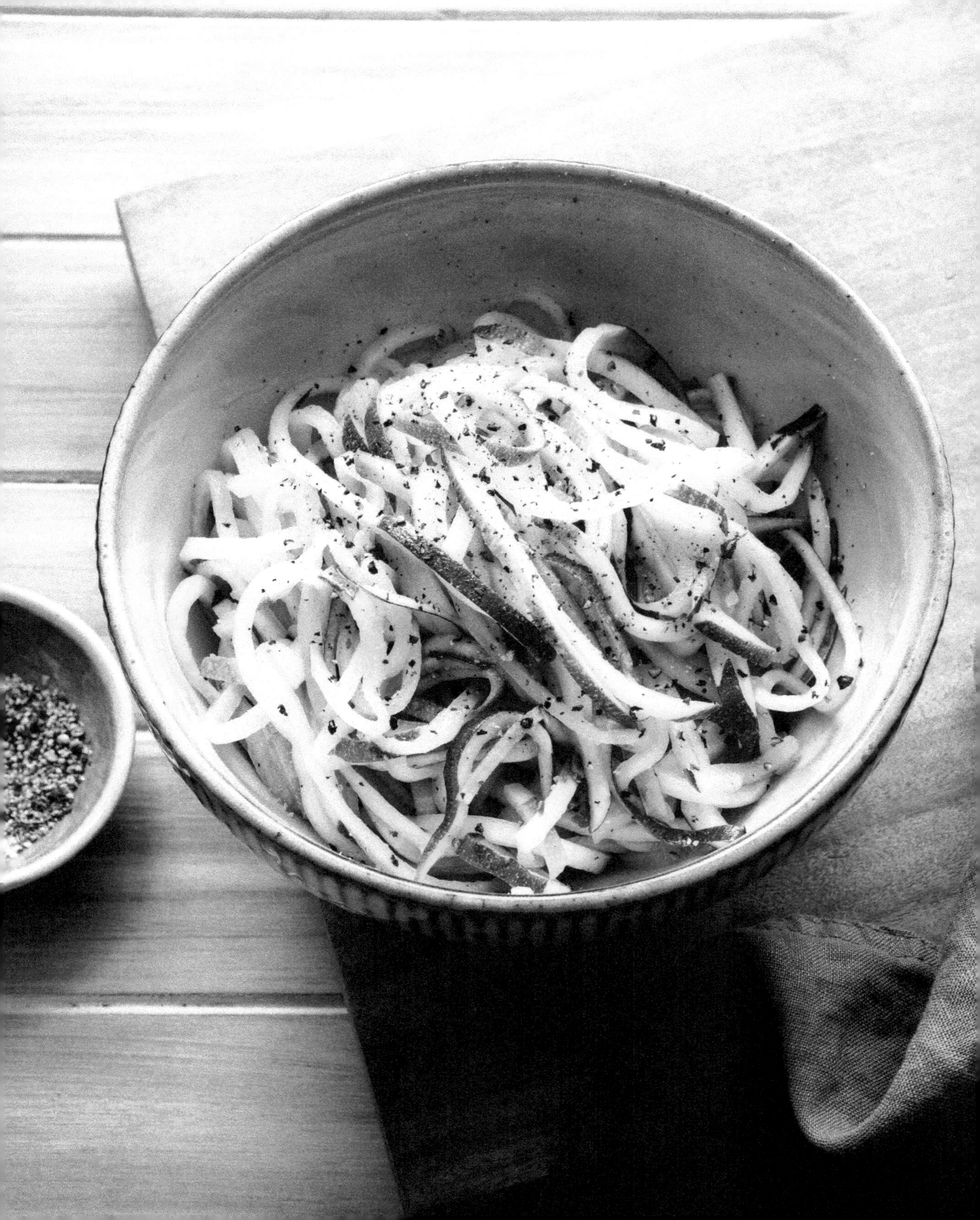

Chapter Two

Basics

(left) Zucchini Noodles

Ghee

Ghee is made by heating butter to separate the milk solids from the fat, and it is a major staple in all of my cooking. It contains lots of beneficial fatty acids, including CLA (conjugated linoleic acid) and butyrate, and it does not contain casein or lactose. Ghee also has a high smoke point, which makes it safe to use when cooking at high temperatures. **MAKES ABOUT 1¾ CUPS**

1 pound unsalted grass-fed butter

1. Select the pressure cooker's Sauté or Browning feature and adjust the heat to medium. Add the butter and cook until the milk solids separate, about 7 to 10 minutes, stirring every few minutes. After cooking, turn off the pressure cooker and let the ghee cool for about 5 to 10 minutes.
2. Set a fine-mesh strainer or cheesecloth and a funnel over a glass jar, and strain the ghee into the jar. Cover and close the jar tightly. Store the ghee in a cool place for up to 3 months or in the refrigerator for up to a year.

COOKING TIP: Cooking time will vary depending on the quality and temperature of the butter and the temperature of the pressure cooker. Click Cancel once the butter is clear and the milk solids have settled on the bottom. The ghee will continue to cook after you press Cancel, and the milk solids should turn brown.

PREP
1 minute

SAUTÉ
11 minutes

TOTAL
12 minutes

- GLUTEN-FREE
- NUT-FREE
- VEGETARIAN

PER SERVING (1 TABLESPOON)
Calories: 120; Total fat: 14g; Total carbs: 0g; Net carbs: 0g; Fiber: 0g; Sugar: 0g; Protein: 0g

MACROS
100% fat
0% carbs
0% protein

Bone Broth

Bone broth is a major staple in my diet. I drink it straight, use it as a substitute for water or stock to cook soups and stews, and use it to add moisture to my cauliflower rice. I love it not only because of its flavor but also because of its amazing health benefits. Bone broth is packed full of minerals, protein, gelatin, and collagen. It has been shown to improve gut health, cushion joints, boost the immune system, and improve the condition of skin and hair. **SERVES 10 TO 12**

2½ pounds assorted combination of organic chicken or beef bones

1 onion, peeled and halved

2 carrots, chopped

2 celery stalks, chopped

5 garlic cloves, peeled

2 or 3 herb sprigs (rosemary, sage, parsley, thyme)

1 tablespoon apple cider vinegar

2 teaspoons pink Himalayan sea salt

½ teaspoon whole black peppercorns

1. Preheat the oven to 450°F.
2. On a rimmed baking sheet, arrange the bones in a single layer and roast for 30 to 35 minutes.
3. Transfer the bones to the pressure cooker. Add the onion, carrots, celery, garlic, herb sprigs, apple cider vinegar, salt, and peppercorns. Cover with water until the pressure cooker is two-thirds full.
4. Lock the lid into place and set the steam release knob to the sealed position. Set the pressure level to High and the time to 120 minutes. After cooking, let the pressure release naturally. Unlock and remove the lid.
5. Set a cheesecloth-lined colander or strainer over a large bowl or pot and strain the broth, discarding the bones and vegetables. Enjoy immediately or let the broth cool and store in tightly closed mason jars for up to 5 days in the refrigerator.

PREP
10 minutes

ROAST
30 minutes

PRESSURE COOK
2 hours on High

RELEASE
Natural

TOTAL
3 hours 30 minutes

- DAIRY-FREE
- GLUTEN-FREE
- NUT-FREE

PER SERVING
Calories: 57; Total fat: 2g; Total carbs: 1g; Net carbs: 1g; Fiber: 0g; Sugar: 0g; Protein: 5g

MACROS
37% fat
41% carbs
22% protein

INGREDIENT TIP: When cooking whole chicken, chicken thighs, or bone-in beef, save and freeze the bones to use for bone broth.

Sugar-Free Sweetened Condensed Milk

This condensed milk is so yummy, I could eat it with a spoon! But I usually resist and use this recipe in some of my favorite desserts, including my pressure cooker Key Lime Pie (page 156). The amount of sweetened condensed milk this recipe produces will vary slightly depending on how much it is reduced while cooking. **MAKES ABOUT 1½ CUPS**

3 cups heavy cream

3 tablespoons unsalted grass-fed butter

½ teaspoon liquid stevia or preferred powdered sugar substitute equivalent to ⅓ cup sugar

1. In a saucepan, combine the heavy cream, butter, and stevia and bring to a boil. After the cream begins to boil, reduce the heat and simmer for 15 to 20 minutes, stirring frequently.
2. When the cream mixture turns a golden brown and has a thick consistency, remove from the heat, let cool, and transfer to an airtight glass jar. Store refrigerated for 3 to 5 days.

PREP
5 minutes

COOK
25 minutes

TOTAL
30 minutes

- GLUTEN-FREE
- NUT-FREE
- VEGETARIAN

PER SERVING (¼ CUP)
Calories: 461; Total fat: 50g; Total carbs: 3g; Net carbs: 3g; Fiber: 0g; Sugar: 3g; Protein: 2g

MACROS
95% fat
3% carbs
2% protein

Avocado Oil Mayonnaise

Mayonnaise is such a wonderful and versatile ingredient. However, conventional mayonnaise is made with unwanted inflammation-causing oils such as canola. This recipe uses olive oil or avocado oil to ensure that you are getting only healthy sources of fat. Add garlic or fresh herbs to this recipe to make delicious variations. **MAKES 1¼ CUPS**

- 2 large egg yolks, at room temperature
- 1 tablespoon freshly squeezed lemon juice
- 1 teaspoon apple cider vinegar
- 1 teaspoon Dijon mustard
- 1 teaspoon sea salt
- 1 cup avocado oil or light olive oil

1. In a food processor, combine the egg yolks, lemon juice, apple cider vinegar, Dijon mustard, and salt. Blend for 20 to 30 seconds.
2. With the food processor running, slowly pour in the oil in a thin stream. Continue to mix until all the oil has been added and the mayonnaise has set.
3. Transfer to an airtight glass jar and store for up to 5 days in the refrigerator.

INGREDIENT TIP: If you don't have avocado oil, mayonnaise is the only time I suggest using light olive oil instead of a higher-quality extra-virgin olive oil. I find the flavor of extra-virgin olive oil too strong for mayonnaise.

PREP
10 minutes, plus 30 minutes to chill

TOTAL
40 minutes

- DAIRY-FREE
- GLUTEN-FREE
- NUT-FREE
- VEGETARIAN

PER SERVING (1 TABLESPOON)
Calories: 105; Total fat: 12g; Total carbs: 0g; Net carbs: 0g; Fiber: 0g; Sugar: 0g; Protein: 0g

MACROS
99% fat
0% carbs
1% protein

Dairy-Free Sour Cream

Because I try to limit dairy in my diet, I have found other ways to up my fat intake by making things like sour cream from coconut milk. I love to pair this recipe with Three-Meat Chili (page 80), Crispy Pork Carnitas (page 144), and Mole Chicken (page 116). **MAKES ¾ CUP**

1 (13.5-ounce) can full-fat coconut milk or ¾ cup full-fat coconut cream

1 tablespoon freshly squeezed lemon juice

1 teaspoon onion powder

⅛ teaspoon sea salt, plus more for seasoning

1 teaspoon chopped chives

PREP
5 minutes

TOTAL
5 minutes

- DAIRY-FREE
- GLUTEN-FREE
- NUT-FREE
- VEGAN

1. If using coconut milk, refrigerate the can for at least 6 hours. This will cause the cream to separate. Open the can of coconut milk and scrape out only the cream into a medium bowl. If using coconut cream, measure out ¾ cup and put it in the bowl.
2. Whisk in the lemon juice, onion powder, sea salt, and chives just until the mixture is well combined and it reaches the desired consistency. Season with additional salt if desired.

PER SERVING
Calories: 45; Total fat: 5g; Total carbs: 1g; Net carbs: 1g; Fiber: 0g; Sugar: 1g; Protein: 1g

MACROS
90% fat
5% carbs
5% protein

Avocado Ranch Dressing

Most store-bought salad dressings are full of unwanted sugars and inflammation-causing oils. This homemade ranch dressing is the perfect substitute because it is full of healthy fats and fresh herbs. **MAKES 1¼ CUPS**

1 avocado, halved, pitted, peeled, and chopped

⅓ cup full-fat coconut cream

⅓ cup Avocado Oil Mayonnaise (page 21)

2 garlic cloves, peeled

2 teaspoons freshly squeezed lemon juice

1 tablespoon chopped fresh dill

2 tablespoons chopped fresh parsley

1 tablespoon chopped fresh chives

1 teaspoon onion powder

1 teaspoon sea salt

½ teaspoon freshly ground black pepper

1. In a blender, combine all of the ingredients. Blend for 1 to 2 minutes, or until smooth.
2. Chill for 1 to 2 hours in the refrigerator. The dressing can be stored in an airtight jar in the refrigerator for up to 1 week.

PREP
5 minutes

TOTAL
8 minutes, plus 1 to 2 hours to chill

- DAIRY-FREE
- GLUTEN-FREE
- NUT-FREE
- VEGETARIAN

PER SERVING
Calories: 68 Total fat: 6g; Total carbs: 3g; Net carbs: 1g; Fiber: 2g; Sugar: 1g; Protein: 1g

MACROS
79% fat
17% carbs
4% protein

Bolognese Sauce

Pancetta, ground beef, and ground pork combine in this Bolognese sauce to create a party in your mouth! By using the pressure cooker, you can save time and effort without sacrificing the amazing depth of flavors you get when you cook the sauce for hours. **SERVES 6**

- 4 ounces pancetta, chopped
- 1 tablespoon unsalted grass-fed butter
- 5 garlic cloves, minced
- 1 large onion, minced
- 1 large celery stalk, minced
- 1 large carrot, minced
- 1 pound ground pork
- 1 pound grass-fed ground beef
- ⅓ cup red wine
- 1 tablespoon balsamic vinegar
- 1 (28-ounce) can crushed tomatoes with their juices
- ½ cup Bone Broth (page 19) or beef broth
- 3 bay leaves
- 1 teaspoon dried oregano
- 1 teaspoon dried basil
- 1 teaspoon sea salt
- ½ teaspoon freshly ground black pepper
- ½ cup heavy cream
- ½ cup freshly grated Parmesan cheese
- ½ cup chopped fresh basil

PREP
8 minutes

SAUTÉ
11 minutes

PRESSURE COOK
15 minutes on High

RELEASE
Natural

TOTAL
1 hour

- GLUTEN-FREE
- NUT-FREE

PER SERVING
Calories: 464; Total fat: 31g; Total carbs: 8g; Net carbs: 6g; Fiber: 2g; Sugar: 4g; Protein: 30g

MACROS
65% fat
7% carbs
28% protein

1. Select the pressure cooker's Sauté or Browning feature and adjust the heat to low. Put the pancetta in the cooker and sauté for 4 to 6 minutes, or until browned.
2. Add the butter, garlic, onion, celery, and carrot and cook for 6 to 8 minutes, or until the vegetables are soft.
3. Add the pork and beef to the pressure cooker and sauté until the meat begins to brown. Use a wooden spoon to break up the meat into small pieces. Add the red wine and balsamic vinegar and continue to sauté for 2 to 3 minutes.

4. Add the tomatoes and their juices, the broth, bay leaves, oregano, dried basil, salt, and pepper. Stir until well mixed, scraping up any browned bits stuck to the bottom of the pan.
5. Lock the lid into place and set the steam release knob to the sealed position. Set the pressure level to High and the time to 15 minutes. After cooking, let the pressure release naturally. Unlock and remove the lid.
6. Switch back to the Sauté function. Stir in the cream, Parmesan cheese, and fresh basil and sauté until the sauce begins to thicken. Remove the bay leaves and serve the sauce over Zucchini Noodles (page 29) or Spaghetti Squash (page 32).

Sugar-Free Barbecue Sauce

Conventional barbecue sauces are full of carbs and sugars, but this simple recipe is sweet, smoky, tangy, and still low-carb. **MAKES 1½ CUPS**

- 10 ounces canned tomato paste
- ¼ cup apple cider vinegar
- 2 tablespoons unsalted grass-fed butter
- 1 tablespoon Worcestershire sauce
- 1 tablespoon garlic powder
- 1 tablespoon onion powder
- 1 teaspoon sea salt
- 1 teaspoon smoked paprika
- ¼ to ½ teaspoon cayenne pepper
- ½ teaspoon chili powder
- 1 teaspoon liquid smoke
- 1 tablespoon Dijon mustard
- ⅓ teaspoon liquid stevia or sugar substitute equivalent to ⅓ cup sugar

1. In a small saucepan, whisk together ½ cup water with the tomato paste, apple cider vinegar, butter, Worcestershire sauce, garlic powder, onion powder, salt, smoked paprika, cayenne, chili powder, liquid smoke, Dijon mustard, and stevia. Bring to a boil, reduce the heat, and simmer for 15 minutes, stirring occasionally. When the sauce reaches the desired consistency, remove from the heat.
2. Let the sauce cool slightly and taste. If needed, adjust the spice and sweetness to your taste by adding more cayenne or stevia. Transfer to an airtight glass storage jar and refrigerate for up to 2 weeks.

PREP
5 minutes

COOK
20 minutes

TOTAL
25 minutes

- GLUTEN-FREE
- NUT-FREE

PER SERVING
Calories: 52; Total fat: 3g; Total carbs: 6g; Net carbs: 1g; Fiber: 5g; Sugar: 3g; Protein: 2g

MACROS
48% fat
41% carbs
11% protein

Guacamole

Avocados are one of my all-time favorite foods. I rarely go a day without eating an entire avocado, and several days a week I have two. If I am not eating them straight with a spoon, I am eating them in this guacamole recipe. **MAKES 3 CUPS**

6 ripe avocados, halved and pitted

Juice of 3 limes

½ onion, minced

¼ cup chopped fresh cilantro

1 garlic clove, minced

½ jalapeño pepper, seeded and minced

½ teaspoon ground cumin

¼ teaspoon ground cayenne pepper

Sea salt

Freshly ground black pepper

1 tablespoon extra-virgin olive oil

1. Scoop out the flesh of the avocados into a mixing bowl. Add the lime juice, onion, cilantro, garlic, jalapeño, cumin, and cayenne. Season with salt and pepper. Use a fork to mash to the desired consistency.
2. Drizzle the guacamole with the olive oil before serving.

INGREDIENT TIP: What are the two most marketed keto foods? Avocado and bacon. Why not put them together? If I am feeling fancy, I add three pieces of cooked crumbled bacon to this guacamole.

TOTAL
10 minutes

- DAIRY-FREE
- GLUTEN-FREE
- NUT-FREE
- VEGAN

PER SERVING (¼ CUP)
Calories: 133; Total fat: 12g; Total carbs: 8g; Net carbs: 3g; Fiber: 5g; Sugar: 1g; Protein: 2g

MACROS
74% fat
22% carbs
4% protein

Hard-boiled and Soft-boiled Eggs

Easy to peel and easy to cook, hard-boiled eggs are a staple in my diet when I am super busy. They are the perfect on-the-go whole-food snack. I will eat them by themselves, or I love to combine them with half an avocado, sea salt, and pepper for a yummy and healthy egg salad. **SERVES 6**

6 large eggs

1. Pour 1 cup of water into the pressure cooker and place the trivet inside. Carefully arrange the eggs on the trivet.
2. Lock the lid into place and set the steam release knob to the sealed position. Set the pressure level to High and the time to 5 minutes for hard-boiled eggs or 2 to 3 minutes for soft-boiled eggs.
3. While the eggs are cooking, fill a medium bowl with water and 3 to 4 ice cubes. After cooking, quick release the pressure. Unlock and remove the lid and carefully transfer the eggs to the ice bath to stop them from overcooking.
4. Once the eggs have cooled, peel and eat them, or store in their shells in the refrigerator for up to one week.

COOKING TIP: Cooking time will vary slightly based on the freshness of the eggs and the altitude.

PREP
1 minute

PRESSURE COOK
5 minutes on High for hard-boiled; 2 to 3 minutes on High for soft-boiled

RELEASE
Quick

TOTAL
16 minutes

- DAIRY-FREE
- GLUTEN-FREE
- NUT-FREE
- VEGETARIAN

PER SERVING
Calories: 71; Total fat: 5g; Total carbs: 0g; Net carbs: 0g; Fiber: 0g; Sugar: 0g; Protein: 6g

MACROS
63% fat
2% carbs
35% protein

Zucchini Noodles

Zucchini noodles, or zoodles, are the perfect pasta substitute and the perfect base for so many recipes. My favorite pairings are the Perfect Italian Meatballs (page 128) or Shrimp Scampi (page 94). **SERVES 4**

2 medium zucchini

2 tablespoons Ghee (page 18)

½ teaspoon sea salt

½ teaspoon freshly ground black pepper

1. Using a knife, spiralizer, or julienne peeler, cut the zucchini into noodle-like strands.
2. In a skillet, melt the ghee over medium heat. Once hot, add the raw zoodles and cook until they soften or reach the desired texture. Season with the salt and pepper and add toppings of your choice.

COOKING TIP: This is my favorite way to prepare zoodles, but they can also be boiled or eaten raw.

PREP
5 minutes

COOK
5 minutes

TOTAL
10 minutes

- GLUTEN-FREE
- NUT-FREE
- VEGETARIAN

PER SERVING
Calories: 75; Total fat: 8g; Total carbs: 2g; Net carbs: 1g; Fiber: 1g; Sugar: 2g; Protein: 0g

MACROS
91% fat
8% carbs
1% protein

Cauliflower Rice Three Ways

Cauliflower rice has become my favorite side dish and a base for both sauces and stews. It is so versatile and can be made with a range of flavor variations. If I am short on time I will often serve it raw, but if time allows, I have included my two favorite variations. **SERVES 4**

BASIC CAULIFLOWER RICE

1 head cauliflower, trimmed

CHEESY CAULIFLOWER RICE

4 tablespoons unsalted grass-fed butter

½ onion, minced

3 garlic cloves, minced

1 recipe Basic Cauliflower Rice

½ cup heavy cream

½ cup chopped fresh basil

½ cup grated Parmesan cheese

¼ cup cream cheese

½ teaspoon onion powder

½ teaspoon sea salt

¼ teaspoon freshly ground black pepper

COCONUT-LIME CAULIFLOWER RICE

4 tablespoons unsalted grass-fed butter

½ onion, minced

3 garlic cloves, minced

1 recipe Basic Cauliflower Rice

¾ cup full-fat coconut milk or heavy cream

Juice of 1 lime

½ teaspoon ground cumin

¼ teaspoon cayenne pepper

¼ cup chopped fresh cilantro

½ teaspoon sea salt

¼ teaspoon freshly ground black pepper

BASIC CAULIFLOWER RICE

PREP
5 minutes

TOTAL
5 minutes

- DAIRY-FREE
- GLUTEN-FREE
- NUT-FREE
- VEGAN

CHEESY CAULIFLOWER RICE AND COCONUT-LIME CAULIFOWER RICE

PREP
5 minutes

COOK
15 minutes

TOTAL
20 minutes

- GLUTEN-FREE
- NUT-FREE
- VEGETARIAN

Basic Cauliflower Rice

Cut the cauliflower into florets and place in a food processor. Pulse until the cauliflower is broken down into rice-size pieces. Serve raw.

Cheesy Cauliflower Rice

1. In a large pan, melt the butter over medium heat. Add the onion and garlic and sauté, stirring frequently, until translucent, about 3 to 5 minutes.
2. Add the cauliflower rice and cook for an additional 5 minutes, stirring occasionally.
3. Add the heavy cream, basil, Parmesan, cream cheese, onion powder, salt, and pepper. Cook for 5 to 8 more minutes, stirring frequently, until the cauliflower reaches the desired consistency.

Coconut-Lime Cauliflower Rice

1. In a large pan, melt the butter over medium heat. Add the onion and garlic and sauté, stirring frequently, until translucent, about 3 to 5 minutes.
2. Add the cauliflower rice and cook for an additional 5 minutes, stirring occasionally.
3. Add the coconut milk, lime juice, cumin, cayenne, cilantro, salt, and pepper. Cook for 5 to 8 more minutes, stirring frequently, until the cauliflower reaches the desired consistency.

PREP TIP: If using coconut milk, put the can in the refrigerator for 6 hours or more before using. This will cause the cream to separate from the milk. Open the can of coconut milk and scrape the cream out. This will make much creamier cauliflower rice. Coconut cream is ideal, and my favorite brand is Trader Joe's.

BASIC CAULIFLOWER RICE PER SERVING (½ CUP)
Calories: 52; Total fat: 0g; Total carbs: 10g; Net carbs: 5g; Fiber: 5g; Sugar: 2g; Protein: 4g

MACROS
0% fat
69% carbs
31% protein

CHEESY CAULIFLOWER RICE PER SERVING (½ CUP)
Calories: 241; Total fat: 28g; Total carbs: 11g; Net carbs: 8g; Fiber: 3g; Sugar: 5g; Protein: 9g

MACROS
76% fat
14% carbs
10% protein

COCONUT-LIME CAULIFLOWER RICE PER SERVING (½ CUP)
Calories: 256; Total fat: 23g; Total carbs: 11g; Net carbs: 8g; Fiber: 3g; Sugar: 5g; Protein: 5g

MACROS
77% fat
16% carbs
7% protein

Spaghetti Squash

Spaghetti squash cooks in a fraction of the time when using a pressure cooker, and it is the perfect low-carb substitute for noodles. Serve this recipe as a healthy side dish or as a base for your protein. **SERVES 4**

PREP
3 minutes

PRESSURE COOK
7 minutes on High

RELEASE
Quick

TOTAL
20 minutes

- GLUTEN-FREE
- NUT-FREE
- VEGETARIAN

1 medium spaghetti squash

Sea salt

Freshly ground black pepper

¼ cup unsalted grass-fed butter, melted

1. Cut the spaghetti squash in half and use a spoon to scoop out the seeds.
2. Pour 1 cup of water into the pressure cooker and place a trivet inside. Place the squash on the trivet.
3. Lock the lid into place and set the steam release knob to the sealed position. Set the pressure level to High and the time to 7 minutes. After cooking, quick release the pressure. Unlock and remove the lid.
4. Using tongs, carefully remove the squash. Use two forks to remove the flesh of the squash and shred it into long strings.
5. Season with salt and pepper and drizzle with the butter.

PER SERVING
Calories: 144; Total fat: 12g; Total carbs: 10g; Net carbs: 7g; Fiber: 3g; Sugar: 4g; Protein: 1g

MACROS
71% fat
26% carbs
3% protein

Simple Shredded Chicken

I meal-prep chicken thighs weekly in my Instant Pot. Shredded chicken thighs are the perfect staple to have on hand to create quick and easy meals. I add the shredded chicken to salads and stir-fries, or simply top it with some Guacamole (page 27) and Avocado Ranch Dressing (page 23) for a five-minute meal. I prefer to prep chicken thighs instead of breasts because thighs are naturally juicier and have more fat to help me hit my macros. **SERVES 6**

2 pounds boneless chicken thighs

1 teaspoon sea salt

½ teaspoon freshly ground black pepper

1 teaspoon garlic powder

1. Generously season the chicken thighs on both sides with the salt, pepper, and garlic powder.
2. Transfer the chicken thighs to the pressure cooker and add ½ cup water.
3. Lock the lid into place and set the steam release knob to the sealed position. Set the pressure level to High and the time to 13 minutes. After cooking, quick release the pressure. Unlock and remove the lid.
4. Carefully remove the chicken and shred with two forks. Transfer to an airtight glass storage container and store refrigerated for 3 to 4 days, or freeze for 2 to 4 months.

PREP
2 minutes

PRESSURE COOK
13 minutes on High

RELEASE
Quick

TOTAL
25 minutes

- DAIRY-FREE
- GLUTEN-FREE
- NUT-FREE

PER SERVING
Calories: 178; Total fat: 6g; Total carbs: 1g; Net carbs: 1g; Fiber: 0g; Sugar: 0g; Protein: 30g

MACROS
31% fat
3% carbs
67% protein

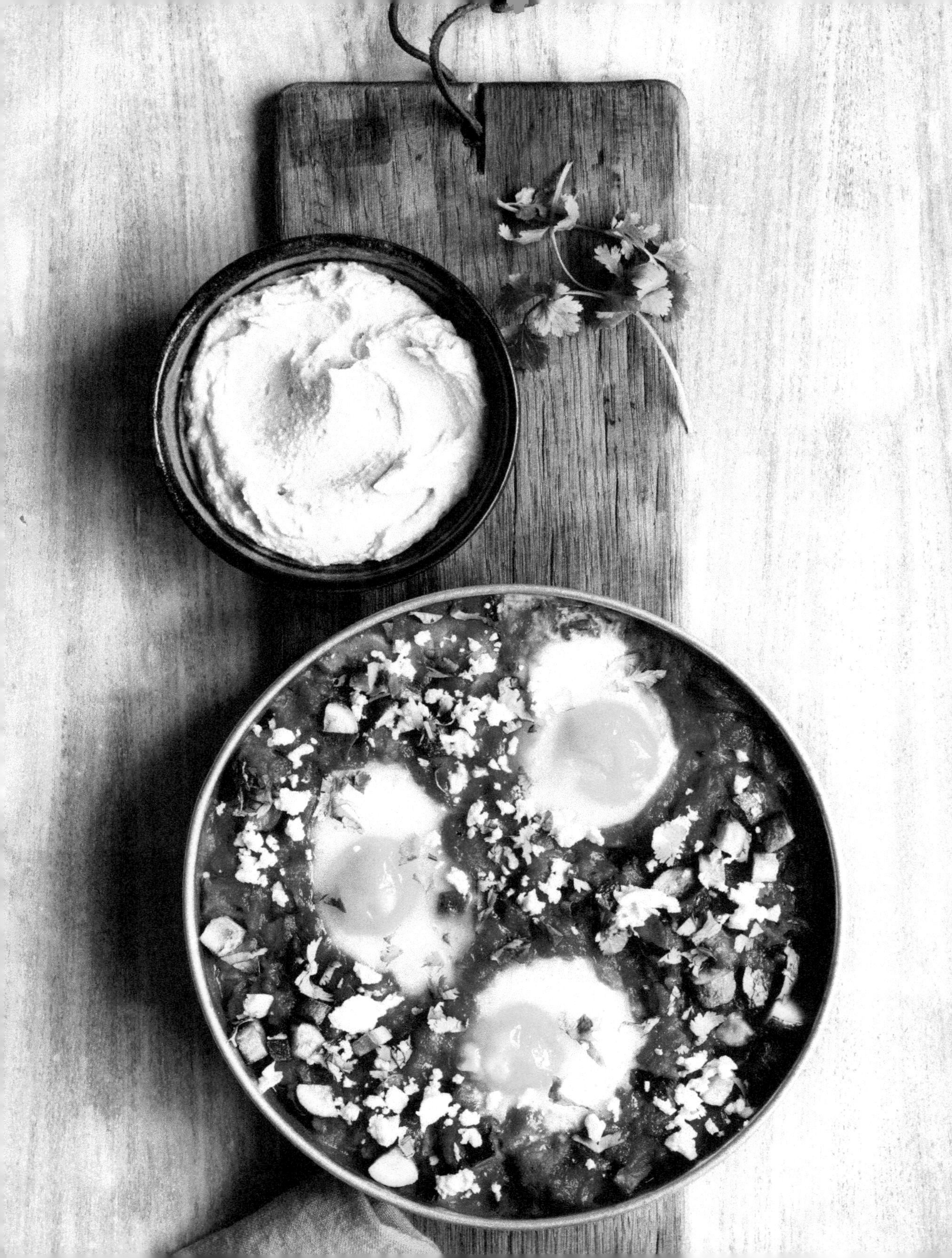

Chapter Three

Breakfast

(left) Shakshuka

Coconut Yogurt

Yogurt was one of my favorite snacks before I started following a ketogenic diet. Most yogurts are too high in carbohydrates and sugar to be eaten on a ketogenic diet. Also, I often limit my dairy consumption due to the inflammation response it causes my body. This recipe lets me eat low-carb and low-dairy and still enjoy delicious, tart yogurt. Keep in mind that the amount of gelatin used will determine the thickness of the yogurt. **SERVES 4**

2 (13.5-ounce) cans full-fat coconut cream

4 high-quality probiotic capsules

2 to 3 teaspoons grass-fed gelatin

1 teaspoon vanilla extract

Stevia (optional)

1. Put the coconut cream in the pressure cooker. Lock the lid into place and set the steam release knob to the open or venting position. Press the yogurt function button and adjust to the Boil setting. Once complete, unlock and remove the lid.
2. Remove the cooker pot from the pressure cooker and let the coconut cream cool until it reaches 100°F to 115°F. Open and empty the contents of the probiotic capsules into the coconut cream, discarding the empty capsules. Whisk together until combined.
3. Return the pot to the pressure cooker, press the yogurt button again, and adjust the setting back to normal. Set the time to 10 to 12 hours. The longer the yogurt incubates, the tarter it will become.

PREP
2 minutes

COOK
About 30 minutes

INCUBATION
10 to 12 hours

TOTAL
12 hours 32 minutes, plus 4 to 6 hours to chill

- DAIRY-FREE
- GLUTEN-FREE
- NUT-FREE

PER SERVING
Calories: 251; Total fat: 23g; Total carbs: 3g; Net carbs: 3g; Fiber: 0g; Sugar: 0g; Protein: 8g

MACROS
83% fat
4% carbs
13% protein

4. When the incubation time is complete, unlock the lid and remove the inner pot of the pressure cooker. Pour the yogurt into a blender or food processor. In a small bowl, mix the gelatin with 3 to 4 tablespoons cold water and mix well. Let sit for 1 minute to bloom. Add the gelatin mixture, vanilla, and stevia (if using) to the blender. Blend until well combined.
5. Let the yogurt cool, then pour into glass containers, close with a tight-fitting lid, and store in the refrigerator for 4 to 6 hours before enjoying. The yogurt may separate when cooled, so stir to combine if necessary. Store in the refrigerator for up to 1 week.

Shakshuka

Shakshuka is a staple in North African and Arab cuisines and one of my favorite pressure cooker recipes. This dish consists of eggs cooked in tomato sauce loaded with spices and topped with hummus and fresh crumbled feta cheese.

SERVES 4

3 tablespoons avocado oil

1 onion, diced

4 garlic cloves, minced

½ medium zucchini, diced

1 teaspoon chili powder

1 teaspoon paprika

1 teaspoon ground cumin

¼ cup Bone Broth (page 19) or chicken broth

2 (14.5-ounce) cans diced tomatoes with their juices

6 large eggs

5 ounces crumbled feta cheese

4 tablespoons hummus

¼ cup chopped fresh cilantro

PREP
3 minutes

SAUTÉ
8 minutes

PRESSURE COOK
0 minutes on Low

RELEASE
Quick

TOTAL
22 minutes

- GLUTEN-FREE
- NUT-FREE

PER SERVING
Calories: 378; Total fat: 26g; Total carbs: 15g; Net carbs: 12g; Fiber: 3g; Sugar: 8g; Protein: 18g

MACROS
64% fat
16% carbs
20% protein

1. Select the pressure cooker's Sauté or Browning feature and adjust the heat to medium. Heat the avocado oil in the cooker until shimmering. Add the onion and garlic and sauté for 3 to 5 minutes, or until fragrant and translucent. Add the zucchini, chili powder, paprika, and cumin and continue to sauté for 1 to 2 minutes.
2. Turn off the pressure cooker and add the bone broth and diced tomatoes and their juices. Stir until everything is mixed. Carefully crack the eggs into the tomato mixture, spacing them evenly and trying not to break the yolks.

3. Lock the lid into place and set the steam release knob to the sealed position. Set the pressure level to Low and the time to 0 minutes. (If you can't set your pressure cooker for 0 minutes, set it for 1 minute, but release the pressure as soon as the pot starts to count down.) After cooking, quick release the pressure. Unlock and remove the lid.
4. Using a ladle, spoon off some of the liquid that has accumulated on top of the eggs. Let cool slightly before serving. Top with the crumbled feta cheese, hummus, and cilantro.

Egg Bites

These egg cups are the perfect meal to prep ahead for a busy week. They are so easy to make, and I often double the recipe and make two batches. Switch up the ingredients with any low-carb vegetables or cheeses to create different flavor combinations. **SERVES 4**

2 tablespoons Ghee (page 18) or oil

4 large eggs

¼ cup heavy cream

½ cup shredded Cheddar cheese, divided

½ teaspoon hot sauce (optional)

½ teaspoon sea salt

¼ teaspoon freshly ground black pepper

4 pieces cooked uncured bacon, crumbled

½ cup chopped baby spinach

PREP
5 minutes

PRESSURE COOK
5 minutes on High

RELEASE
Quick

TOTAL
20 minutes

- GLUTEN-FREE
- NUT-FREE

PER SERVING
Calories: 230; Total fat: 19g; Total carbs: 2g; Net carbs: 2g; Fiber: 0g; Sugar: 2g; Protein: 13g

MACROS
76% fat
4% carbs
20% protein

1. Grease four ovenproof custard cups or wide-mouth half-pint jars with the ghee.
2. In a large bowl, whisk the eggs, cream, ¼ cup of cheese, hot sauce (if using), salt, and pepper until just blended. Evenly divide the bacon and spinach among the prepared custard cups or jars. Pour the egg mixture over the bacon and spinach. Cover each custard cup or jar loosely with aluminum foil.
3. Pour 1 cup of water into the pressure cooker and place a trivet inside. Place the custard cups or jars on the trivet. It's okay to stack them if they don't fit in one layer.

4. Lock the lid into place and set the steam release knob to the sealed position. Set the pressure level to High and the time to 5 minutes. After cooking, quick release the pressure. Unlock and remove the lid.
5. Carefully remove the custard cups or jars from the pressure cooker. Discard the foil and sprinkle with the remaining ¼ cup of cheese.

PREP TIP: I recently purchased large silicone muffin cups and love making this recipe in them!

Avocado Eggs Benedict

Eggs Benedict has been a favorite of mine since I was a child, and this keto variation never disappoints. I have swapped out the bread for sliced avocado and the Canadian bacon for uncured bacon, but you could also use low-carb biscuits and Canadian bacon if you are craving something more traditional.

SERVES 4

- 1 tablespoon avocado oil
- 4 large eggs, plus 2 large egg yolks
- 1 tablespoon freshly squeezed lemon juice
- ¼ teaspoon sea salt, plus more for seasoning
- ¼ teaspoon paprika
- ¼ teaspoon cayenne pepper
- 4 tablespoons unsalted grass-fed butter, melted
- 2 avocados, pitted, peeled, and sliced
- 4 slices cooked uncured bacon
- Freshly ground black pepper

1. Grease four silicone cups with the avocado oil. Crack each whole egg into a prepared silicone cup.
2. Pour 1 cup of water into the pressure cooker and place a trivet inside. Carefully place the egg cups on the trivet. Lock the lid into place and set the steam release knob to the sealed position. Set the cooker on Steam for 2 to 3 minutes on High.
3. While the eggs are cooking, in a blender, combine the egg yolks, lemon juice, salt, paprika, and cayenne. Blend for 5 to 10 seconds, or until combined.
4. Set the blender on high speed and pour in the hot melted butter in a thin stream. The mixture should thicken quickly. Set the blender jar in a pan of hot tap water to keep the hollandaise sauce warm until serving.

PREP
5 minutes

STEAM
3 minutes on High

RELEASE
Natural for 3 minutes, then Quick

TOTAL
15 minutes

- GLUTEN-FREE
- NUT-FREE

PER SERVING
Calories: 393; Total fat: 35g; Total carbs: 8g; Net carbs: 3g; Fiber: 5g; Sugar: 2g; Protein: 13g

MACROS
79% fat
8% carbs
13% protein

5. When the pressure cooking time is complete, let the pressure release naturally for 3 minutes, then quick release any remaining pressure. Carefully remove the silicone cups from the pressure cooker.
6. Divide the avocado slices among four plates and top with the cooked bacon and poached eggs. Pour the hollandaise sauce over the top and season with salt and pepper.

COOKING TIP: When poaching eggs, I have noticed different results with the same cook time depending on the temperature of the water and the freshness of the eggs. Typically, 2 to 3 minutes results in perfectly poached eggs.

Eggs Florentine

Eggs Florentine is a wonderful twist on traditional eggs Benedict, using spinach in place of Canadian bacon. This elegant and delicious meal is done in just 30 minutes. **SERVES 4**

3 tablespoons Ghee (page 18), divided

1 small onion, chopped

1 pound spinach

1 teaspoon sea salt, divided

4 tablespoons cream cheese, softened and cut into 6 to 8 small pieces

½ cup heavy cream

4 large eggs

Freshly ground black pepper

PREP
5 minutes

SAUTÉ
12 minutes

PRESSURE COOK
3 minutes on High

RELEASE
Quick

TOTAL
30 minutes

- GLUTEN-FREE
- NUT-FREE
- VEGETARIAN

PER SERVING
Calories: 360; Total fat: 33g; Total carbs: 8g; Net carbs: 5g; Fiber: 3g; Sugar: 4g; Protein: 11g

MACROS
79% fat
9% carbs
12% protein

1. Select the pressure cooker's Sauté or Browning feature and adjust the heat to medium. Heat 2 tablespoons of ghee in the cooker until shimmering. Add the onion and cook, stirring, for 2 to 3 minutes, until softened slightly. Add the spinach in big handfuls, stirring to wilt before adding the next handful. When all the spinach is wilted, add ½ teaspoon of the salt and stir. There will probably be some liquid in the bottom of the pot; blot it out with paper towels or carefully pour it out.
2. Add the cream cheese and heavy cream to the spinach and stir until the cream cheese melts and the heavy cream thickens, about 4 minutes.
3. Divide the spinach mixture evenly among four small ramekins or custard cups, using a spoon to push it up the sides to create a well in the middle. Crack one egg into each cup and sprinkle with the remaining ½ teaspoon of salt and pepper. Divide the remaining 1 tablespoon of ghee into four small pieces and place one on top of each egg. Cover the cups with aluminum foil, crimping it down.

4. Wipe out the pressure cooker, pour in 1½ cups water, and place a trivet inside. Carefully place the egg cups onto the trivet, stacking them if necessary to fit.
5. Lock the lid into place and set the steam release knob to the sealed position. Set the pressure level to High and the time to 3 minutes. After cooking, quick release the pressure. Unlock but don't remove the lid. Let the eggs sit in the pressure cooker for 30 seconds before removing the lid; this will help ensure that the whites are fully cooked. Use tongs to remove the cups from the cooker and remove the foil. Let cool for a few minutes before serving.

INGREDIENT TIP: You may find spinach packaged in 9- or 10-ounce bags. If so, use two full bags if you like, leaving the rest of the recipe as is; you'll just have extra spinach in the cups.

Scotch Eggs

Traditional Scotch eggs have an outside coating of bread crumbs, but you can leave them off for a keto version and still have a delicious snack or breakfast. Feel free to use any bulk sausage you like in place of the breakfast sausage.

SERVES 4

4 large eggs

¾ pound bulk breakfast sausage

¼ cup avocado oil

1. Pour 1¾ cups water into the pressure cooker and place a trivet inside. Carefully arrange the eggs on the trivet. Prepare an ice bath by filling a medium bowl half full with cold water and adding a handful of ice cubes.
2. Lock the pressure cooker lid into place and set the steam release knob to the sealed position. Set the pressure level to High and the time to 3 minutes. After cooking, quick release the pressure. Unlock and remove the lid.
3. Using tongs, transfer the eggs to the ice bath and let cool for 3 to 4 minutes or until cool enough to handle. Carefully peel the eggs and blot them dry.
4. Divide the sausage into four pieces and flatten each piece into an oval. One at a time, place an egg on a sausage oval and carefully pull the sausage around the egg, sealing the edges.

PREP
10 minutes

SAUTÉ
15 minutes

PRESSURE COOK
3 minutes on High

RELEASE
Quick

TOTAL
40 minutes

- DAIRY-FREE
- GLUTEN-FREE
- NUT-FREE

PER SERVING
Calories: 482; Total fat: 44g; Total carbs: 2g; Net carbs: 2g; Fiber: 0g; Sugar: 1g; Protein: 17g

MACROS
84% fat
2% carbs
14% protein

5. Pour the water out of the pressure cooker pot and dry the pot. Select the Sauté or Browning feature, adjust the heat to medium, and heat the avocado oil in the cooker until shimmering. Add the sausage-wrapped eggs and cook for 1 to 2 minutes, then turn the eggs to cook on the other side for a couple of minutes. When the sausage is completely browned on all sides, remove one egg and test the sausage with the tip of a knife to make sure it's cooked through. If not, return to the pot and cook for another few minutes until done. Transfer the eggs to a rack and let cool for a few minutes before serving.

Breakfast Crustless Quiche

This one-pot breakfast quiche couldn't be easier to make than when using a pressure cooker. This delicious dish is perfect for weekend brunch with the family or prepared ahead of time and used for breakfast on-the-go on busy weekday mornings. It combines healthy greens, savory sausage, fluffy eggs, and a little kick of feta for a mouthwatering and whole-food-based breakfast delight. **SERVES 4**

2 tablespoons Ghee (page 18) or preferred cooking oil, divided

6 ounces ground sausage

2 tablespoons minced onion

1 teaspoon minced garlic

1 cup chopped kale

¼ cup chopped fresh chives

8 large eggs

¼ cup heavy cream

1 teaspoon sea salt

½ teaspoon freshly ground black pepper

½ cup crumbled feta cheese, divided

PREP
7 minutes

SAUTÉ
8 minutes

PRESSURE COOK
25 minutes on High

RELEASE
Natural for 10 minutes, then Quick

TOTAL
1 hour

- GLUTEN-FREE
- NUT-FREE

PER SERVING
Calories: 524; Total fat: 41g; Total carbs: 5g; Net carbs: 4g; Fiber: 1g; Sugar: 2g; Protein: 33g

MACROS
71% fat
4% carbs
25% protein

1. Select the pressure cooker's Sauté or Browning feature and adjust the heat to medium. Heat 1 tablespoon of ghee in the cooker, add the sausage, and sauté, stirring often, for 4 to 5 minutes, or until browned. Add the onion and garlic and cook until the onion becomes translucent. Stir in the kale and chives. Transfer the mixture to a plate, set aside, and wipe the pot clean.
2. In a medium bowl, whisk together the eggs and cream until combined. Stir in the salt and pepper and set aside.
3. Grease a 7-inch springform pan or baking dish with the remaining 1 tablespoon of ghee. Spoon the sausage mixture into the pan. Pour the egg mixture over the sausage. Top with ¼ cup of feta cheese and cover with aluminum foil.

4. Pour 2 cups of water into the pressure cooker and place a trivet inside. Place the springform pan on the trivet. If the trivet does not have handles, create a foil sling to lower the pan onto the trivet (see Prep Tip).
5. Close and lock the lid and set the steam release knob to the sealed position. Set the pressure level to High and the time to 25 minutes. After cooking, let the pressure release naturally for 10 minutes, then quick release any remaining pressure. Unlock and remove the lid. Using the trivet's handles or the foil sling, remove the pan from the pressure cooker.
6. Using a knife, slide around the outside of the pan to remove any egg mixture stuck to the pan. Remove the outer ring of the pan. Sprinkle the remaining ¼ cup of feta cheese on top of the quiche and serve.

PREP TIP: Create a sling out of aluminum foil by folding it lengthwise in thirds and wrapping it around the bottom of the springform pan.

Southwestern Breakfast Casserole

Spicy green chiles and Mexican chorizo are balanced out with rich cream and Monterey Jack cheese. My cheesy breakfast casserole is hearty enough for brunch, lunch, or even dinner! **SERVES 6**

- 4 large eggs
- ½ cup heavy cream
- ½ cup half-and-half
- ½ teaspoon sea salt
- ¼ teaspoon freshly ground black pepper
- 1 tablespoon Ghee (page 18)
- 2 (4-ounce) cans whole green chiles, drained and blotted dry
- 4 ounces Monterey Jack or other mild cheese, grated (about 2½ cups), divided
- 1 pound crumbled cooked Mexican chorizo, divided

1. In a medium bowl, whisk the eggs well. Add the cream, half-and-half, salt, and pepper and whisk to combine.
2. Coat the bottom and sides of a 1½-quart baking dish with the ghee. Split the chiles open and place enough of them in the bottom of the dish to form a single layer. Sprinkle one-third of the cheese over the chiles, then top with half of the chorizo. Top with another layer of chiles, then add another third of the cheese, reserving the last third. Top with the remaining chorizo. If you have more chiles left, add another layer (it's fine if you don't).
3. Carefully pour the egg mixture over the casserole. You may not need all of it; fill the dish to about ½ inch from the top. Cover the dish with aluminum foil. Do not crimp it down as the casserole will expand; you just want to keep moisture off the top.

PREP
10 minutes

PRESSURE COOK
12 minutes on High

RELEASE
Natural for 10 minutes, then Quick

TOTAL
40 minutes

- GLUTEN-FREE
- NUT-FREE

PER SERVING
Calories: 582; Total fat: 50g; Total carbs: 4; Net carbs: 4g; Fiber: 0g; Sugar: 1g; Protein: 27g

MACROS
78% fat
3% carbs
19% protein

4. Pour 1½ cups of water into the pressure cooker and place a trivet with handles inside. Place the casserole on top of the trivet. If your trivet doesn't have handles, use a foil sling (page 49) to make removing the bowl easier.
5. Lock the lid into place and set the steam release knob to the sealed position. Set the pressure level to High and the time to 12 minutes. After cooking, let the pressure release naturally for 10 minutes, then quick release any remaining pressure. Unlock and remove the lid.
6. Carefully remove the casserole from the pot. Test it to make sure it's done by inserting a knife in the center; the knife should come out clean. If it does not, return the casserole to the pressure cooker and lock the lid back in place so it finishes cooking, about 5 minutes.
7. Preheat the oven to broil (you can do this while the casserole cooks). Remove the foil and sprinkle the reserved cheese over the top of the casserole. Place the dish under the broiler for 3 to 4 minutes, or until the cheese melts and starts to brown.
8. Let the casserole cool for a few minutes before serving.

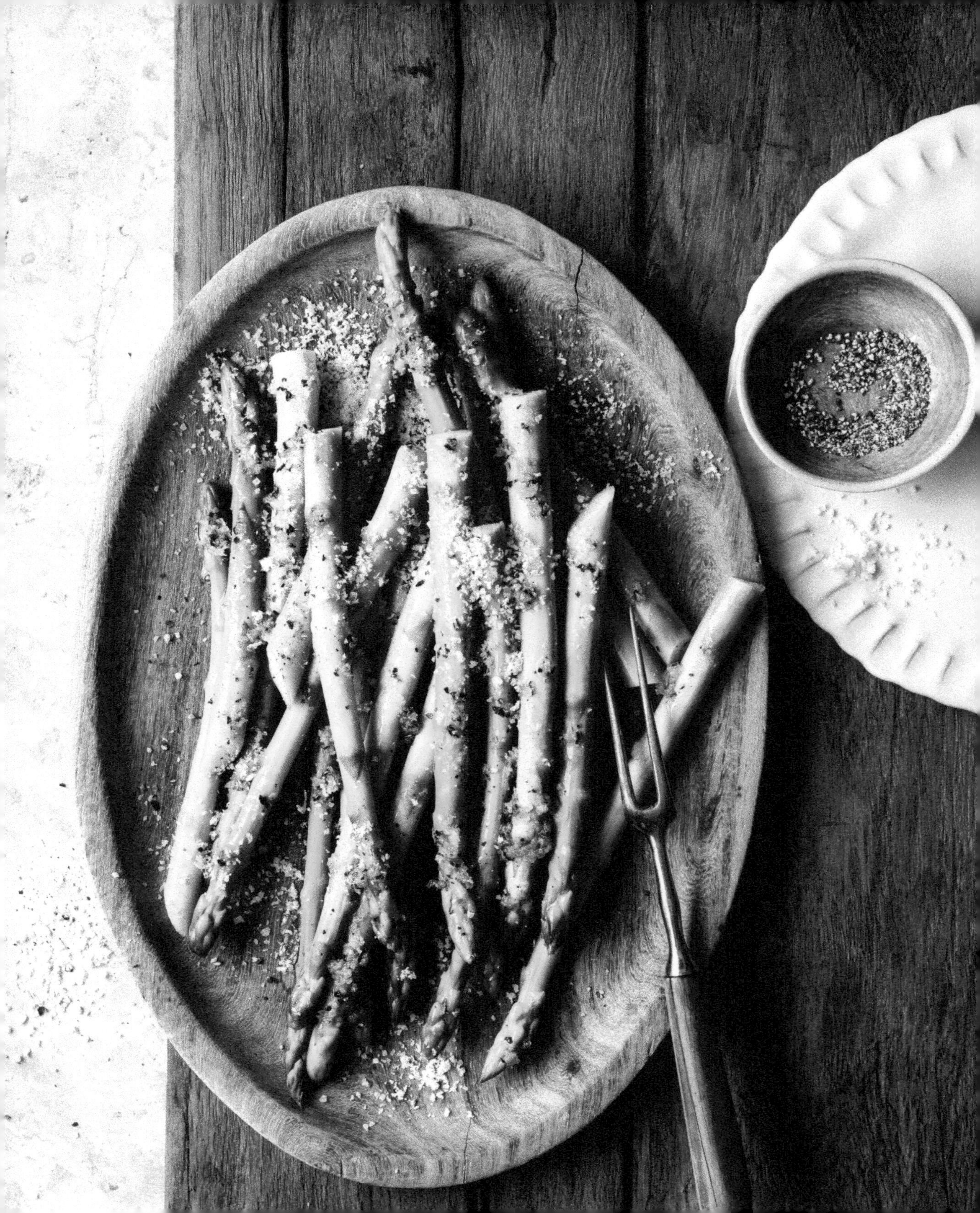

Chapter Four

Vegetables and Sides

(left) Asparagus with Parmesan

Cauliflower Purée

Butter, heavy cream, and Parmesan cheese—do I need to say more? This combination of ingredients makes this cauliflower purée a decadent indulgence. This dish pairs perfectly with Homemade Sliced Turkey and Gravy (page 124) to create a guilt-free, keto-fied Thanksgiving meal. **SERVES 4**

1 large head cauliflower

1 cup Bone Broth (page 19) or chicken broth

4 tablespoons unsalted grass-fed butter, plus more for serving

¼ cup heavy cream

4 garlic cloves, minced

1 cup shredded Parmesan cheese

½ teaspoon sea salt

½ teaspoon freshly ground black pepper

Scallions, green parts only, sliced, for serving

PREP
3 minutes

PRESSURE COOK
3 minutes on High

RELEASE
Quick

FINISHING
3 minutes

TOTAL
20 minutes

- GLUTEN-FREE
- NUT-FREE

PER SERVING
Calories: 295; Total fat: 23g; Total carbs: 10g; Net carbs: 6g; Fiber: 4g; Sugar: 4g; Protein: 12g

MACROS
70% fat
13% carbs
17% protein

1. Remove the core of the cauliflower and roughly chop the cauliflower into chunks.
2. Pour the bone broth into the pressure cooker and place the steamer basket inside. Arrange the cauliflower evenly in the steamer basket.
3. Lock the lid into place and set the steam release knob to the sealed position. Set the pressure level to High and the time to 3 minutes. After cooking, quick release the pressure. Unlock and remove the lid.
4. Transfer the cauliflower to a food processor. Add the 4 tablespoons of butter, the cream, garlic, Parmesan cheese, salt, and pepper. Process until the mixture has reached a smooth consistency.
5. Serve the cauliflower purée with sliced scallions and more butter.

SUBSTITUTION TIP: Make this dish dairy-free by substituting coconut cream for the heavy cream and olive oil for the butter, and eliminating the Parmesan cheese.

Collard Greens

Collard greens are packed full of antioxidants and are high in both vitamins C and K. They are also a great source of fiber, which can often be lacking in a high-fat diet. I have combined the nutritious collard greens with crispy bacon and garlic for a healthy and delectable dish. **SERVES 5**

10 slices thick uncured bacon, chopped

1 onion, sliced

4 garlic cloves, minced

6 cups chopped collard greens

2 cups Bone Broth (page 19) or chicken broth

¼ teaspoon red pepper flakes

1 tablespoon apple cider vinegar

6 to 9 drops liquid stevia or 2 tablespoons sugar substitute

½ teaspoon sea salt

1. Select the pressure cooker's Sauté or Browning feature and adjust the heat to medium. When hot, put in the chopped bacon, onion, and garlic and sauté for about 8 minutes, or until the bacon begins to crisp.
2. Add the collard greens, bone broth, red pepper flakes, apple cider vinegar, stevia, and salt.
3. Lock the lid into place and set the steam release knob to the sealed position. Set the pressure level to High and the time to 20 minutes. After cooking is complete, let the pressure release naturally for 5 minutes, then quick release any remaining pressure. Unlock and remove the lid.
4. Serve the collard greens hot.

PREP
2 minutes

SAUTÉ
8 minutes

PRESSURE COOK
20 minutes on High

RELEASE
Natural for 5 minutes, then Quick

TOTAL
40 minutes

- DAIRY-FREE
- GLUTEN-FREE
- NUT-FREE

PER SERVING
Calories: 221; Total fat: 15g; Total carbs: 4g; Net carbs: 2g; Fiber: 2g; Sugar: 0g; Protein: 15g

MACROS
65% fat
8% carbs
27% protein

Bacon Brussels Sprouts

Bacon adds a wonderful sweetness to the natural bitterness of Brussels sprouts. Combined with almonds and balsamic vinegar, this recipe is the perfect side dish. **SERVES 6**

16 ounces Brussels sprouts, trimmed and halved

6 thick slices uncured bacon, chopped

2 garlic cloves, minced

¼ cup sliced almonds

1 teaspoon onion powder

1 teaspoon red pepper flakes

2 tablespoons balsamic vinegar

½ teaspoon sea salt

1. Pour 2 cups of water into the pressure cooker and place the steamer basket inside. Arrange the Brussels sprouts evenly in the steamer basket.
2. Lock the lid into place and set the steam release knob to the sealed position. Set the pressure level to High and the time to 1 minute. After cooking, quick release the pressure. Unlock and remove the lid.
3. Remove the Brussels sprouts from the pressure cooker. Remove the steamer basket and empty the water from the pressure cooker.
4. Select the pressure cooker's Sauté or Browning feature and adjust the heat to medium. Add the bacon and cook until it is almost crisp. Return the Brussels sprouts to the pressure cooker. Add the garlic, almonds, onion powder, red pepper flakes, balsamic vinegar, and salt. Continue to sauté, stirring occasionally, until the Brussels sprouts are browned and begin to crisp, about 6 to 8 minutes.

PREP
3 minutes

PRESSURE COOK
1 minute on High

RELEASE
Quick

SAUTÉ
8 minutes

TOTAL
25 minutes

- DAIRY-FREE
- GLUTEN-FREE

PER SERVING
Calories: 181; Total fat: 11g; Total carbs: 14g; Net carbs: 9g; Fiber: 5g; Sugar: 4g; Protein: 8g

MACROS
67% fat
12% carbs
21% protein

Asparagus with Parmesan

Asparagus is packed full of vitamins and is high in fiber. The fiber content keeps the net carbs very low, making it a great low-carb vegetable choice. Here, it is topped with a brown butter sauce, making this dish not only nutrient-dense but also high in fat and flavor. **SERVES 4**

- 1 pound asparagus, hard ends trimmed
- 4 tablespoons unsalted grass-fed butter
- 2 garlic cloves, minced
- 1 teaspoon dried basil
- ¼ cup grated Parmesan cheese
- Sea salt
- Freshly ground black pepper

PREP
3 minutes

PRESSURE COOK
0 minutes on High

SAUTÉ
8 minutes

RELEASE
Quick

TOTAL
23 minutes

- GLUTEN-FREE
- NUT-FREE
- VEGETARIAN

PER SERVING
Calories: 231; Total fat: 19g; Total carbs: 6g; Net carbs: 3g; Fiber: 3g; Sugar: 2g; Protein: 12g

MACROS
70% fat
10% carbs
20% protein

1. Pour 1 cup of water into the pressure cooker and place the steaming rack inside. Arrange the asparagus evenly on the steaming rack.
2. Lock the lid into place and set the steam release knob to the sealed position. Set the pressure level to High and the time to 0 minutes. (If you can't set your pressure cooker for 0 minutes, set it for 1 minute, but release the pressure as soon as the pot starts to count down.) After cooking, quick release the pressure. Unlock and remove the lid.
3. Lift the steaming rack out of the pressure cooker and transfer the asparagus to a plate, tenting it with aluminum foil to keep warm. Empty the water from the pressure cooker.
4. Select the Sauté or Browning feature and adjust the heat to high. Combine the butter, garlic, and basil in the pressure cooker. Cook, stirring occasionally, for 6 to 8 minutes, or until the butter is lightly browned.
5. Arrange the asparagus on a serving platter. Pour the butter sauce over the asparagus and sprinkle with Parmesan cheese. Season with salt and pepper.

Lemon-Garlic Broccoli

I always stress to my clients not to overthink cooking keto. Cook green vegetables in yummy fat and seasonings, and you will hit your macro and micro nutrient goals. This recipe is a perfect example of using simple ingredients to create a flavorful and nutrient-dense side dish. **SERVES 5**

4 cups broccoli florets

3 tablespoons unsalted grass-fed butter

4 garlic cloves, chopped

1 tablespoon onion powder

1 teaspoon sea salt

¼ teaspoon red pepper flakes

Juice of ½ lemon

1. Pour 1 cup of water into the pressure cooker, place the steamer basket inside, and arrange the broccoli in the basket.
2. Lock the lid into place and set the steam release knob to the sealed position. Set the pressure level to High and the time to 0 minutes. (If you can't set your pressure cooker for 0 minutes, set it for 1 minute, but release the pressure as soon as the pot starts to count down.) After cooking, quick release the pressure. Unlock and remove the lid.
3. Remove the broccoli from the pressure cooker. Remove the steamer basket and empty the water from the pressure cooker.
4. Select the pressure cooker's Sauté or Browning feature and adjust the heat to medium. Heat the butter in the cooker until foaming. Add the garlic and sauté for 1 to 2 minutes, or until lightly browned. Add the broccoli, onion powder, salt, red pepper flakes, and lemon juice. Mix until the broccoli is evenly coated in butter and seasonings.
5. Transfer the broccoli to a serving dish and drizzle with any butter left inside the pressure cooker.

PREP
5 minutes

PRESSURE COOK
0 minutes on High

RELEASE
Quick

SAUTÉ
3 minutes

TOTAL
20 minutes

- GLUTEN-FREE
- NUT-FREE
- VEGETARIAN

PER SERVING
Calories: 122; Total fat: 9g; Total carbs: 9g; Net carbs: 6g; Fiber: 3g; Sugar: 2g; Protein: 3g

MACROS
62% fat
29% carbs
9% protein

Sweet-and-Sour Cabbage

This cabbage recipe has the tang of apple cider vinegar balanced out with the sweetness of coconut milk and stevia to create a simple but flavorful dish. I like my food spicy, so I have added a kick of red pepper flakes, but feel free to omit that ingredient if you can't take the heat. **SERVES 4**

¼ cup coconut oil

½ onion, minced

4 garlic cloves, minced

1 medium head cabbage, shredded

½ teaspoon red pepper flakes

3 tablespoons apple cider vinegar

1 teaspoon sea salt, plus more for seasoning

1 tablespoon onion powder

¼ cup full-fat coconut milk

6 to 8 drops liquid stevia or preferred powdered sugar substitute equivalent to 1 to 2 tablespoons sugar (optional)

Freshly ground black pepper

PREP
5 minutes

SAUTÉ
3 minutes

PRESSURE COOK
3 minutes on Low

RELEASE
Quick

TOTAL
23 minutes

- DAIRY-FREE
- GLUTEN-FREE
- NUT-FREE
- VEGAN

PER SERVING
Calories: 122; Total fat: 12g; Total carbs: 10g; Net carbs: 4g; Fiber: 3g; Sugar: 9g; Protein: 4g

MACROS
66% fat
24% carbs
10% protein

1. Select the pressure cooker's Sauté or Browning feature and adjust the heat to medium. Heat the coconut oil in the cooker until shimmering. Add the onion and garlic and sauté until the onion becomes translucent.
2. Add the cabbage, red pepper flakes, apple cider vinegar, salt, onion powder, coconut milk, and stevia (if using) and mix well.
3. Lock the lid into place and set the steam release knob to the sealed position. Set the pressure level to Low and the time to 3 minutes. After cooking, quick release the pressure. Unlock and remove the lid. Season with salt and pepper.

COOKING TIP: I prefer my cabbage to have a crunch. If you like it soft, naturally release the pressure for 5 minutes, followed by a quick release.

Parmesan Artichokes and Garlic Aioli

Artichokes are one of my favorite vegetables to cook in a pressure cooker. They always come out wonderfully, and by using the pressure cooker the cooking time is cut way down! Enjoy these artichokes with a garlic aioli or a dipping sauce of your choice. **SERVES 4**

4 medium artichokes

Juice of 1 lemon, divided

¾ cup grated Parmesan cheese

1 teaspoon sea salt, plus more for seasoning

1 teaspoon freshly ground black pepper, plus more for seasoning

¾ cup Avocado Oil Mayonnaise (page 21)

2 garlic cloves, minced

1. Trim 1 inch off the top of the artichokes and drizzle three-quarters of the lemon juice evenly over them. Spread the leaves of the artichokes and sprinkle the Parmesan cheese, 1 teaspoon of salt, and 1 teaspoon of pepper inside the leaves.
2. Pour 1 cup of water into the pressure cooker and place the trivet inside. Arrange the artichokes stem-side down on the trivet.
3. Lock the lid into place and set the steam release knob to the sealed position. Set the pressure level to High and the time to 10 minutes.
4. While the artichokes are cooking, in a small bowl, prepare the dipping sauce by mixing the mayonnaise, garlic, and remaining lemon juice. Season with salt and pepper.
5. After the artichokes are done cooking, quick release the pressure. Unlock and remove the lid.
6. Using tongs, carefully remove the artichokes from the pressure cooker, transfer to plates, and serve with the dipping sauce.

PREP
2 minutes

PRESSURE COOK
10 minutes on High

RELEASE
Quick

TOTAL
22 minutes

- GLUTEN-FREE
- NUT-FREE
- VEGETARIAN

PER SERVING
Calories: 417; Total fat: 35g; Total carbs: 7g; Net carbs: 4g; Fiber: 3g; Sugar: 3g; Protein: 11g

MACROS
81% fat
8% carbs
11% protein

COOKING TIP: Test to see if the artichokes are done by pulling a leaf from the center and tasting it. If it is still hard, lock the pressure cooker lid back into place and cook the artichokes for an additional 2 to 3 minutes on High pressure.

Easy Pesto Spaghetti Squash

This easy and fresh recipe is a wonderful vegetable side or can easily be turned into the main course by topping the squash with a protein dish. My favorite pairings for this dish are the Simple Shredded Chicken (page 33) or Perfect Italian Meatballs (page 128). **SERVES 4**

1 medium spaghetti squash

1 tablespoon Ghee (page 18)

1 onion, diced

½ cup pesto

3 Roma tomatoes, sliced

Sea salt

Freshly ground black pepper

2 teaspoons extra-virgin olive oil

1. Cut the spaghetti squash in half and use a spoon to scoop out the seeds.
2. Pour 1 cup of water into the pressure cooker and place the trivet inside. Place the squash on the trivet, cut-side up.
3. Lock the lid into place and set the steam release knob to the sealed position. Set the pressure level to High and the time to 7 minutes. After cooking, quick release the pressure. Unlock and remove the lid.
4. Remove the squash from the pot. Using two forks, shred the squash into long strings.
5. Remove the trivet and drain the water from the pressure cooker. Select the Sauté or Browning feature and adjust the heat to medium. Add the ghee. When it's shimmering, add the onion and sauté for about 5 minutes, until it becomes translucent.
6. Add the shredded squash, pesto, and tomatoes and continue to sauté for 1 to 2 minutes, or until heated through and mixed. Season with salt and pepper and drizzle with the olive oil.

PREP
3 minutes

PRESSURE COOK
7 minutes on High

RELEASE
Quick

SAUTÉ
7 minutes

TOTAL
27 minutes

- GLUTEN-FREE
- VEGETARIAN

PER SERVING
Calories: 312; Total fat: 25g; Total carbs: 9g; Net carbs: 9g; Fiber: 0g; Sugar: 3g; Protein: 9g

MACROS
76% fat
12% carbs
12% protein

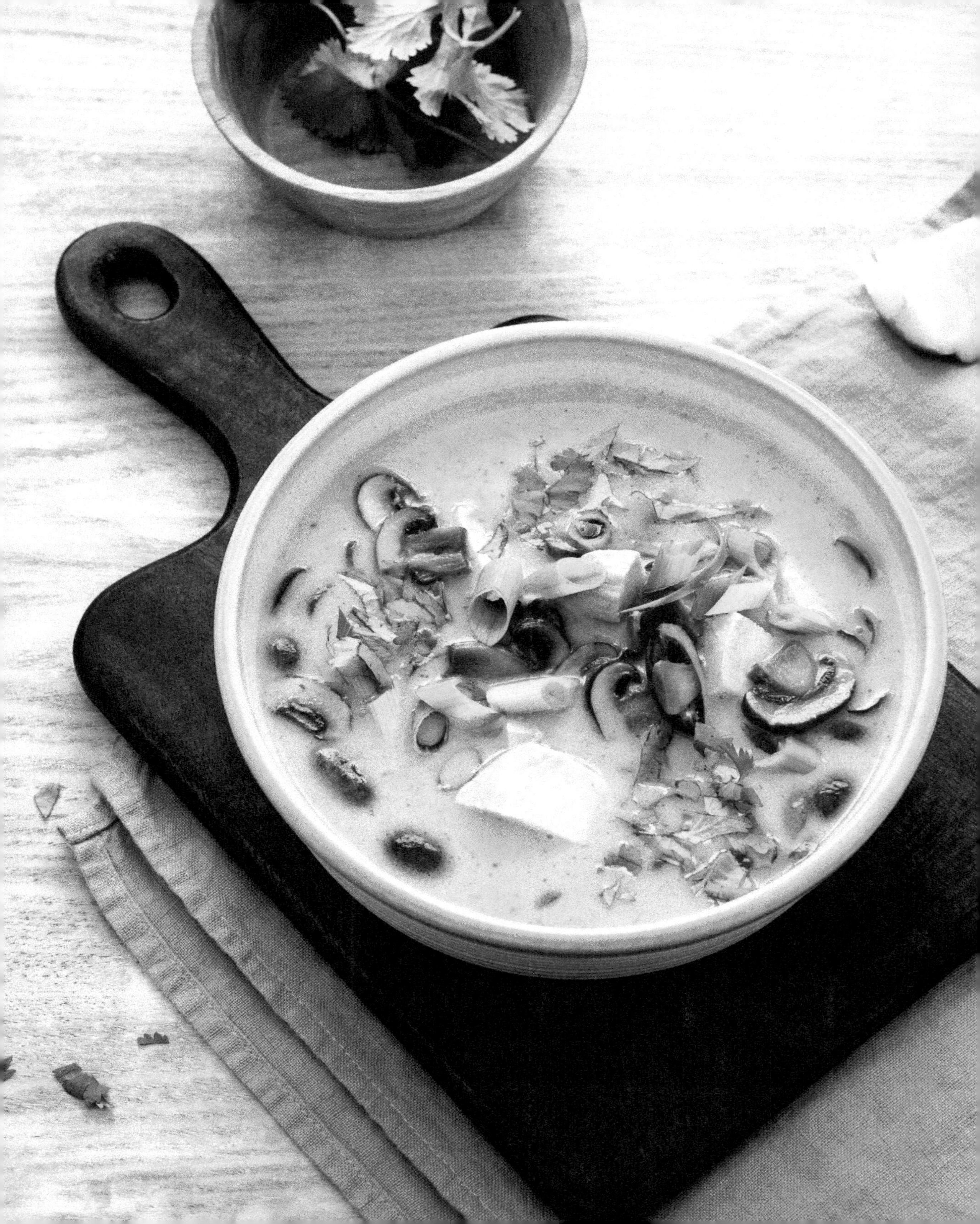

Chapter Five

Soups and Stews

(left) Tom Kha Gai

Roasted Garlic Cauliflower Soup

This is my favorite healing soup when I am feeling under the weather. It's made with ginger, garlic, and turmeric, three superfoods that are packed full of antioxidants and have been shown to have multiple health properties. Enjoy this soup when you need a little extra nutritional boost! **SERVES 4**

- 2 tablespoons avocado oil
- 3 tablespoons Ghee (page 18)
- 1 head garlic, cloves separated and peeled
- 1 onion, diced
- 1 carrot, diced
- 6 cups cauliflower florets
- 4 cups Bone Broth (page 19) or chicken broth
- 1 teaspoon ground turmeric
- 1 teaspoon peeled minced fresh ginger
- 1 teaspoon ground cumin
- 1 teaspoon dried oregano
- 1 teaspoon sea salt
- ¼ teaspoon freshly ground black pepper
- ½ cup full-fat coconut cream
- 3 tablespoons chopped fresh parsley

PREP
5 minutes

SAUTÉ
15 minutes

PRESSURE COOK
8 minutes on High

RELEASE
Quick

TOTAL
30 minutes

- GLUTEN-FREE
- NUT-FREE

PER SERVING
Calories: 370; Total fat: 28g; Total carbs: 15g; Net carbs: 10g; Fiber: 5g; Sugar: 10g; Protein: 18g

MACROS
71% fat
17% carbs
12% protein

1. Select the pressure cooker's Sauté or Browning feature and adjust the heat to low. Put in the avocado oil and ghee and heat until the ghee is melted. Add the garlic and cook, stirring occasionally, until the cloves begin to turn golden brown, about 10 minutes. Add the onion and carrot and sauté for 5 minutes. Add the cauliflower, broth, turmeric, ginger, cumin, oregano, salt, and pepper.
2. Lock the lid into place and set the steam release knob to the sealed position. Set the pressure level to High and the time to 10 minutes. After cooking, quick release the pressure. Unlock and remove the lid.

3. Using an immersion blender, blend the soup until it reaches a smooth consistency. (You can also use a regular blender; be careful to work in batches and hold the lid on. Return the soup to the pressure cooker when done blending.)
4. Divide the soup among four bowls. Stir in the coconut cream and garnish with the parsley.

MACRO TIP: Increase the protein in this soup by topping with some Simple Shredded Chicken (page 33). The macros of this recipe with chicken are 57% fat, 13% carbs, and 30% protein.

No-Noodle Chicken Soup

In this comforting chicken soup, I have replaced noodles with chopped cabbage. I love the texture cabbage creates in the soup, but for a different variation, you can try adding zucchini noodles or spaghetti squash instead. If using frozen chicken, add 10 minutes to the pressure cooking time in step 2. **SERVES 4**

3 tablespoons Ghee (page 18)

4 garlic cloves, minced

1 onion, chopped

1½ pounds boneless, skinless chicken thighs

6 cups Bone Broth (page 19) or chicken broth

3 teaspoons sea salt, plus more for seasoning

1 teaspoon freshly ground black pepper, plus more for seasoning

2 cups chopped cabbage

3 carrots, sliced

4 celery stalks, chopped

2 teaspoons dried thyme

1 teaspoon dried oregano

1 to 2 tablespoons beef gelatin or ¼ to ½ teaspoon xanthan gum

2 teaspoons freshly squeezed lemon juice

PREP
3 minutes

SAUTÉ
5 minutes

PRESSURE COOK
10 minutes on High, plus 2 minutes on High

RELEASE
Quick

TOTAL
30 minutes

- GLUTEN-FREE
- NUT-FREE

PER SERVING
Calories: 482; Total fat: 29g; Total carbs: 12g; Net carbs: 3g; Fiber: 9g; Sugar: 5g; Protein: 48g

MACROS
52% fat
9% carbs
39% protein

1. Select the pressure cooker's Sauté or Browning feature and adjust the heat to medium. Put in the ghee and heat until shimmering. Add the garlic and onion and sauté until the onion becomes translucent, about 5 minutes.
2. Add the chicken, broth, 3 teaspoons of salt, and 1 teaspoon of pepper. Lock the lid into place and set the steam release knob to the sealed position. Set the pressure level to High and the time to 10 minutes. After cooking, quick release the pressure. Unlock and remove the lid.
3. Remove the chicken with a slotted spoon, transfer to a plate, and, using two forks, shred the meat. Return the chicken to the pressure cooker.

4. Add the cabbage, carrots, celery, thyme, and oregano. Lock the lid into place and set the steam release knob to the sealed position. Set the pressure level to High and the time to 2 minutes. After cooking, quick release the pressure. Unlock and remove the lid.
5. To thicken the soup, mix 1 tablespoon of gelatin into a few tablespoons of cool water until dissolved, then let sit for 1 minute. Add to the soup slowly until it reaches the desired consistency (the soup will continue to thicken as it cools), adding more gelatin mixed with water as needed. If using xanthan gum, stir ¼ teaspoon at a time into the soup until it reaches the desired consistency.
6. Add the lemon juice and season the soup with salt and pepper. Divide among four bowls and serve.

Tom Kha Gai

Tom kha gai is a coconut-lime Thai soup. I substituted more commonly accessible foods for some of the traditional ingredients to make it a similar but easier recipe to prepare. If you want to try a more traditional variation, substitute sliced kaffir lime leaves for the lime zest and smashed Thai red chiles for the chili sauce. **SERVES 5**

1½ pounds boneless, skinless chicken breasts

2 cups Bone Broth (page 19) or chicken broth

2 (13.5-ounce) cans full-fat coconut milk

2 lemongrass stalks, tough outer layers removed, chopped into 4-inch pieces

1 tablespoon finely grated lime zest

¼ cup freshly squeezed lime juice

2 tablespoons peeled minced fresh ginger

2 tablespoons fish sauce

2 bay leaves

4 cups sliced mushrooms

1 tablespoon sweet dried basil

1 tablespoon red chili paste

2 scallions, green parts only, sliced

¼ cup chopped fresh cilantro

Sea salt

Freshly ground black pepper

Lime wedges, for serving

PREP
5 minutes

PRESSURE COOK
10 minutes on High

RELEASE
Natural for 10 minutes, then Quick

TOTAL
35 minutes

- DAIRY-FREE
- GLUTEN-FREE
- NUT-FREE

PER SERVING
Calories: 417; Total fat: 29g; Total carbs: 10g; Net carbs: 9g; Fiber: 1g; Sugar: 4g; Protein: 32g

MACROS
61% fat
9% carbs
30% protein

1. In the pressure cooker, combine the chicken, broth, coconut milk, lemongrass, lime zest, lime juice, ginger, fish sauce, bay leaves, mushrooms, basil, chili paste, and scallions and stir well.
2. Lock the lid into place and set the steam release knob to the sealed position. Set the pressure level to High and the time to 10 minutes. After cooking, let the pressure release naturally for 10 minutes, then quick release any remaining pressure. Unlock and remove the lid.
3. Using a slotted spoon, remove and discard the bay leaves and lemongrass. With the slotted spoon, transfer the chicken to a plate and cut into bite-size pieces. Return the chicken to the soup and add the chopped cilantro. Mix well and season with salt and pepper. Serve in soup bowls, with lime wedges.

PREP TIP: When preparing the lemongrass stalks, remove the loose outer layers of leaves. Slice the lower white sections of the lemongrass into 4-inch sections. Before adding them to the soup, use a knife to smash the lemongrass to help release its flavor.

Kale and Sausage Soup

This comforting and yummy soup is full of healthy kale and Italian sausage. If you are dairy-sensitive, the heavy cream can be replaced with coconut milk and the Parmesan cheese can be excluded. **SERVES 5**

1 pound Italian sausage

1 medium onion, minced

6 garlic cloves, minced

1 teaspoon dried oregano

1 cup diced tomatoes

4 cups Bone Broth (page 19) or chicken broth

1 teaspoon sea salt, plus more for seasoning

¼ teaspoon freshly ground black pepper, plus more for seasoning

6 cups chopped kale

1 cup heavy cream or full-fat coconut milk

½ cup grated Parmesan cheese

PREP
5 minutes

SAUTÉ
5 minutes

PRESSURE COOK
5 minutes on High

RELEASE
Natural for 10 minutes, then Quick

TOTAL
35 minutes

- GLUTEN-FREE
- NUT-FREE

PER SERVING
Calories: 523; Total fat: 37g; Total carbs: 15g; Net carbs: 10g; Fiber: 5g; Sugar: 6g; Protein: 27g

MACROS
67% fat
12% carbs
21% protein

1. Select the pressure cooker's Sauté or Browning feature and adjust the heat to medium. Put in the sausage and use a wooden spoon to crumble the meat. Add the onion, garlic, oregano, tomatoes, broth, 1 teaspoon of salt, and ¼ teaspoon of pepper. Cook until the onions are translucent and the sausage is browned, about 5 minutes.
2. Lock the lid into place and set the steam release knob to the sealed position. Set the pressure level to High and the time to 5 minutes. After cooking, let the pressure release naturally for 10 minutes, then quick release any remaining pressure. Unlock and remove the lid.
3. Stir in the kale, cream, and Parmesan cheese. Continue to stir until the kale softens. Season with more salt and pepper. Divide among bowls and serve.

Beef Stew

Hearty beef stew is the quintessential comfort food. I used to make a variation of this recipe in a slow cooker and it would need to cook all day. This delicious pressure cooker version is done in just an hour. **SERVES 6**

2 pounds grass-fed chuck roast or beef brisket, cut into 2-inch chunks

2 teaspoons coarse sea salt, divided

1 teaspoon freshly ground black pepper, plus more for seasoning

3 tablespoons avocado oil

2 onions, sliced

1 pound mushrooms, quartered

6 garlic cloves, sliced

2 tablespoons tomato paste

¾ cup red wine

1 teaspoon dried thyme

1 teaspoon dried oregano

2 bay leaves

½ cup Bone Broth (page 19) or beef broth

¼ cup chopped fresh parsley

PREP
10 minutes

SAUTÉ
5 minutes

PRESSURE COOK
35 minutes on High

RELEASE
Quick

TOTAL
1 hour

- DAIRY-FREE
- GLUTEN-FREE
- NUT-FREE

1. In a large bowl, toss the beef with 1½ teaspoons of coarse sea salt and 1 teaspoon of pepper. Set aside.
2. Select the pressure cooker's Sauté or Browning feature and adjust the heat to medium. Heat the avocado oil in the cooker until shimmering. Once the oil is hot, add the onions, mushrooms, and garlic. Cook, stirring occasionally, for about 5 minutes, or until the onions become translucent. Add the tomato paste, red wine, beef, thyme, oregano, bay leaves, and broth and mix well.
3. Lock the lid into place and set the steam release knob to the sealed position. Set the pressure level to High and the time to 35 minutes. After cooking, quick release the pressure. Unlock and remove the lid.
4. Remove the bay leaves and season the stew with the remaining ½ teaspoon of salt and more pepper. Serve in bowls, garnished with the chopped parsley.

PER SERVING
Calories: 509; Total fat: 33g; Total carbs: 8g; Net carbs: 5g; Fiber: 3g; Sugar: 2g; Protein: 32g

MACROS
65% fat
7% carbs
28% protein

INGREDIENT SUBSTITUTION: For a variation on this recipe, add carrots or celery after the beef is done cooking. Relock the lid into place and cook on High pressure for 5 more minutes.

Pumpkin-Coconut Soup

Okay, call me basic... but just because I follow a ketogenic or low-carb diet doesn't mean I want to miss out on all things pumpkin! Where I grew up in Utah, fall is my favorite time of year, and this soup is my favorite fall dish. Pumpkin is higher in carbs, so watch your serving size on this recipe. **SERVES 5**

2 tablespoons coconut oil

1 onion, diced

4 garlic cloves, minced

1 tablespoon peeled minced fresh ginger

1 teaspoon curry powder

2 teaspoons ground cinnamon

1 teaspoon ground nutmeg

½ teaspoon ground cloves

2 teaspoons sea salt, plus more for seasoning

½ teaspoon freshly ground black pepper, plus more for seasoning

2 cups pumpkin purée

2 cups Bone Broth (page 19) or chicken broth

1 (13.5-ounce) can full-fat coconut cream

1 tablespoon freshly squeezed lime juice

4 to 6 drops liquid stevia or preferred powdered sugar substitute equivalent to 1 to 2 teaspoons sugar (optional)

¼ cup toasted pumpkin seeds

¼ cup chopped fresh cilantro

PREP
3 minutes

SAUTÉ
5 minutes

PRESSURE COOK
10 minutes on High

RELEASE
Natural for 10 minutes, then Quick

TOTAL
38 minutes

- DAIRY-FREE
- GLUTEN-FREE
- NUT-FREE

PER SERVING
Calories: 215; Total fat: 16g; Total carbs: 13g; Net carbs: 2g; Fiber: 11g; Sugar: 6g; Protein: 5g

MACROS
67% fat
25% carbs
8% protein

1. Select the pressure cooker's Sauté or Browning feature and adjust the heat to medium. Heat the coconut oil in the cooker until shimmering. Add the onion and cook for 4 to 5 minutes, until tender. Add the garlic and ginger and cook, stirring, for about 1 minute, or until fragrant.

2. Stir in the curry powder, cinnamon, nutmeg, cloves, 2 teaspoons of salt, and ½ teaspoon of pepper. Add the pumpkin purée and broth and whisk until well mixed.

3. Lock the lid into place and set the steam release knob to the sealed position. Set the pressure level to High and the time to 10 minutes. After cooking, let the pressure release naturally for 10 minutes, then quick release any remaining pressure. Unlock and remove the lid.
4. Use an immersion blender or transfer the soup to a blender and blend until smooth. If using a traditional blender, transfer the soup back to the pressure cooker.
5. Switch the pressure cooker back to the Sauté or Browning setting. Add the coconut cream, lime juice, and stevia (if using), and stir until well mixed and heated through. Season with more salt and pepper.
6. Serve the soup in bowls, garnished with the toasted pumpkin seeds and cilantro.

Roasted Tomato Soup

This is my absolute favorite summertime soup. Ideally, I make it with fresh ingredients straight from my own garden. There is nothing as delicious as a bowl of fresh tomato-basil soup made from homegrown tomatoes, basil, and garlic. **SERVES 5**

- 3 pounds Roma tomatoes, cut lengthwise
- 2 tablespoons avocado oil
- Sea salt
- Freshly ground black pepper
- 3 tablespoons unsalted grass-fed butter
- 1 head garlic, cloves separated and peeled
- 1 yellow onion, minced
- 1 medium carrot, shredded
- 2 cups Bone Broth (page 19) or chicken broth
- 2 tablespoons coconut aminos
- ¼ cup oil-packed sun-dried tomatoes, drained and chopped
- 1 cup chopped fresh basil
- 1 teaspoon dried thyme
- ½ cup heavy cream
- ½ cup cream cheese

PREP
5 minutes

SAUTÉ
12 minutes

PRESSURE COOK
3 minutes on High

RELEASE
Natural for 10 minutes, then Quick

TOTAL
45 minutes

- GLUTEN-FREE
- NUT-FREE

PER SERVING
Calories: 317; Total fat: 24g; Total carbs: 13g; Net carbs: 8g; Fiber: 5g; Sugar: 5g; Protein: 7g

MACROS
73% fat
17% carbs
10% protein

1. Preheat the oven to broil.
2. On a baking sheet, arrange the tomatoes cut-side up. Drizzle with the avocado oil and season with salt and pepper. Place the tomatoes as close as possible to the broiler element and cook for 3 to 5 minutes, or until blackened in spots. Remove from the oven and let cool slightly.
3. Meanwhile, select the pressure cooker's Sauté or Browning feature, adjust the heat to medium, and melt the butter in the cooker until foaming. Add the garlic cloves and cook for 4 to 5 minutes, or until starting to turn golden brown. Add the onion and carrot and sauté for 3 to 4 minutes.

4. Add the broth, coconut aminos, sun-dried tomatoes, basil, thyme, and the roasted tomatoes.
5. Lock the lid into place and set the pressure level to high and the time to 3 minutes. After cooking, allow the pressure to naturally release for 10 minutes, then quick release any remaining pressure.
6. Using an immersion blender, blend the soup until smooth. Alternatively, transfer the soup to a blender in small batches and blend until smooth, then transfer the soup back to the pressure cooker.
7. Add the heavy cream and cream cheese and stir until the cream cheese is melted. Season with salt and pepper and serve in bowls.

COOKING TIP: If tomatoes are not in season, add 1 to 2 tablespoons powdered sugar substitute or 6 to 8 drops liquid stevia to balance out the acidity.

Vietnamese Zoodle Pho

Pho is a delicious Vietnamese dish, and by replacing the traditional rice noodles with zoodles, it becomes keto-friendly. Each bowl gets constructed individually with zoodles and thin slices of beef. Steaming-hot broth is then poured over the top to cook both the beef and zoodles. Enjoy this dish with a variety of delicious toppings. **SERVES 4**

FOR THE BROTH

8 cups Bone Broth (page 19)

2 large onions, cut into quarters

1 tablespoon coconut aminos

1 tablespoon fish sauce

2 cinnamon sticks

3 whole cloves

4 tablespoons peeled sliced fresh ginger

FOR THE PHO

12 ounces sirloin steak

3 cups spiralized zucchini noodles (zoodles)

2 cups bean sprouts

1 jalapeño pepper, thinly sliced

½ cup chopped fresh basil

¼ cup chopped fresh mint

¼ cup chopped fresh cilantro

2 scallions, green parts only, sliced

2 tablespoons fish sauce

2 limes, cut into wedges

Hot sauce (optional)

PREP
2 minutes

PRESSURE COOK
10 minutes on High

RELEASE
Quick

TOTAL
22 minutes

- DAIRY-FREE
- GLUTEN-FREE
- NUT-FREE

PER SERVING
Calories: 257; Total fat: 19g; Total carbs: 15g; Net carbs: 10g; Fiber: 5g; Sugar: 5g; Protein: 22g

MACROS
54% fat
19% carbs
27% protein

To make the broth

1. In the pressure cooker, combine the bone broth, onions, coconut aminos, fish sauce, cinnamon sticks, cloves, and ginger. Lock the lid into place and set the steam release knob to the sealed position. Set the pressure level to High and the time to 10 minutes. After cooking, quick release the pressure. Unlock and remove the lid.
2. Using a fine-mesh strainer or cheesecloth, strain the broth into another pot or large bowl.

To make the pho

1. While the broth is cooking, very thinly slice the steak against the grain. Divide the zoodles among four bowls and evenly divide the steak slices on top.
2. Immediately ladle the steaming broth into each bowl. The beef should start to turn opaque. To serve, top with the bean sprouts, jalapeño slices, basil, mint, cilantro, and scallions, and garnish with the fish sauce, lime wedges, and hot sauce (if using).
3. If you are not going to use the broth immediately, pour it back into the pressure cooker and use the Sauté or Browning feature to bring it to a simmer before using. It's important that the broth be hot in order to cook the beef.

PREP TIP: Freeze the meat for 15 minutes before cutting to make slicing it thinly easier.

Hungarian Mushroom Soup

Keep warm and cozy on a cold winter night by serving this delicious soup. This creamy, savory recipe is the perfect keto-friendly comfort food. **SERVES 4**

- 3 tablespoons unsalted grass-fed butter
- 2 cups sliced onions
- 3 garlic cloves, minced
- 1 pound mushrooms, sliced
- 1 teaspoon sea salt
- 2 cups Bone Broth (page 19) or chicken broth
- ½ cup dry white wine
- 2 teaspoons dried dill weed
- 1 tablespoon paprika
- 1 tablespoon coconut aminos
- ½ cup heavy cream
- 2 teaspoons freshly squeezed lemon juice
- ¼ cup chopped fresh parsley
- ½ cup sour cream
- Freshly ground black pepper

1. Select the pressure cooker's Sauté or Browning feature and adjust the heat to medium. Melt the butter in the cooker until foaming. Add the onions and garlic and sauté for 3 to 5 minutes, or until the onions become translucent. Add the mushrooms and salt and sauté for 5 more minutes. Remove ½ cup of mushrooms and set aside.
2. Add the broth, wine, dill, paprika, and coconut aminos to the cooker and mix well.
3. Lock the lid into place and set the steam release knob to the sealed position. Set the pressure level to High and the time to 20 minutes. After cooking, quick release the pressure. Unlock and remove the lid.

PREP
5 minutes

SAUTÉ
10 minutes

PRESSURE COOK
20 minutes on High

RELEASE
Quick

TOTAL
55 minutes

- GLUTEN-FREE
- NUT-FREE

PER SERVING
Calories: 331; Total fat: 18.5g; Total carbs: 15g; Net carbs: 12g; Fiber: 3g; Sugar: 7g; Protein: 8g

MACROS
72% fat
18% carbs
10% protein

4. Use an immersion blender or transfer the soup to a blender and blend until smooth. Add the heavy cream and continue to blend until well mixed. If using a traditional blender, transfer the soup back to the pressure cooker.
5. Add the lemon juice, parsley, reserved ½ cup of mushrooms, and the sour cream. Mix well and season with pepper. Divide the soup among bowls and serve.

INGREDIENT SUBSTITUTION: Going dairy-free? Replace the sour cream with Dairy-Free Sour Cream (page 22), and use coconut cream in place of the heavy cream.

Three-Meat Chili

This chili is a meat-lover's dream. It combines beef, bacon, and sausage to create a hearty and flavorful meal. Pair it with fresh sliced avocado and coconut cream to keep this dish dairy-free. **SERVES 6**

1 pound uncured bacon, chopped

5 garlic cloves, minced

2 yellow onions, diced

1 green bell pepper, diced

1 pound grass-fed ground beef

1 pound hot Italian sausage

2 (14.5-ounce) cans diced tomatoes with their juices

1 (8-ounce) can tomato paste

1 tablespoon chili powder

1 tablespoon smoked paprika

1 tablespoon ground cumin

1 cup Bone Broth (page 19) or beef broth

¼ cup chopped fresh cilantro

1 avocado, halved, pitted, peeled, and sliced

⅓ cup full-fat coconut cream

PREP
5 minutes

SAUTÉ
10 minutes

PRESSURE COOK
30 minutes on High

RELEASE
Quick

TOTAL
55 minutes

- DAIRY-FREE
- GLUTEN-FREE
- NUT-FREE

PER SERVING
Calories: 612; Total fat: 45g; Total carbs: 16g; Net carbs: 12g; Fiber: 3g; Sugar: 6g; Protein: 33g

MACROS
68% fat
10% carbs
22% protein

1. Select the pressure cooker's Sauté or Browning feature and adjust the heat to medium. Put in the bacon and cook, stirring, until crisp. Use a slotted spoon to remove the bacon, leaving the fat behind.
2. Add the garlic, onions, and green pepper to the cooker and sauté in the bacon fat for 3 to 5 minutes. Add the beef, sausage, diced tomatoes and their juices, tomato paste, chili powder, smoked paprika, cumin, and bone broth. Cook, stirring occasionally, for 3 to 5 minutes.

3. Return the bacon to the pressure cooker. Lock the lid into place and set the steam release knob to the sealed position. Set the pressure level to High and the time to 30 minutes. After cooking, quick release the pressure. Unlock and remove the lid.
4. Divide the chili among bowls and serve garnished with the chopped cilantro, avocado slices, and coconut cream.

INGREDIENT SUBSTITUTION: I often remove dairy from my diet because I find it very inflammatory for my body. Coconut cream and coconut milk can be used in almost any recipe to replace cream, milk, or sour cream. If you're not dairy-free, top the chili with sour cream and shredded cheese.

White Chicken Chili

Creamy white chicken chili was a favorite of mine growing up. This low-carb take on my childhood favorite is just as delicious as I remember. This soup is for the lover of all things dairy. It is made with heavy cream, cream cheese, and sour cream, and topped with shredded cheese! **SERVES 6**

- 2 tablespoons unsalted grass-fed butter
- 1 onion, diced
- 4 garlic cloves, minced
- 1½ pounds boneless, skinless chicken thighs
- 1 (4-ounce) can green chiles
- 1 teaspoon chili powder
- 1 teaspoon ground cumin
- 1 teaspoon dried oregano
- 2 teaspoons sea salt
- 1 teaspoon freshly ground black pepper
- 3 cups Bone Broth (page 19) or chicken broth
- ½ cup heavy cream
- ½ cup cream cheese
- ½ cup sour cream
- 2 avocados, halved, pitted, peeled, and diced
- ½ cup shredded Cheddar cheese
- ¼ cup chopped fresh cilantro
- 1 lime, cut into wedges

PREP
5 minutes

SAUTÉ
8 minutes

PRESSURE COOK
10 minutes on High

RELEASE
Natural for 10 minutes, then Quick

TOTAL
42 minutes

- GLUTEN-FREE
- NUT-FREE

PER SERVING
Calories: 509; Total fat: 37g; Total carbs: 11g; Net carbs: 7g; Fiber: 4g; Sugar: 4g; Protein: 30g

MACROS
67% fat
8% carbs
25% protein

1. Select the pressure cooker's Sauté or Browning feature and adjust the heat to medium. Melt the butter in the cooker until foaming. Add the onion and garlic and sauté for about 4 minutes, or until the onion becomes translucent.
2. Add the chicken and brown for 2 to 3 minutes on each side. Add the chiles, chili powder, cumin, oregano, salt, pepper, and broth.

3. Lock the lid into place and set the steam release knob to the sealed position. Set the pressure level to High and the time to 10 minutes. After cooking, let the pressure release naturally for 10 minutes, then quick release any remaining pressure. Unlock and remove the lid. Using a slotted spoon, transfer the chicken thighs to a plate. Using two forks, shred the meat, then transfer back to the pressure cooker.
4. Add the heavy cream, cream cheese, and sour cream. Mix until the cream cheese melts.
5. Serve the chili in bowls, topped with the diced avocado, shredded cheese, chopped cilantro, and lime wedges.

Chunky Clam Chowder

Just because you are eating a ketogenic diet doesn't mean you can't enjoy a creamy bowl of clam chowder! This recipe is so simple using a pressure cooker, and it's done in about 30 minutes. **SERVES 8**

6 slices bacon, chopped

6 garlic cloves, minced

1 onion, diced

2 cups chopped celery

2 pounds frozen cauliflower florets

5 (6.5-ounce) cans chopped clams, drained

1 (8-ounce) bottle clam juice

2 cups Bone Broth (page 19) or chicken broth

1 tablespoon dried thyme

1 teaspoon sea salt, plus more for seasoning

½ teaspoon freshly ground black pepper, plus more for seasoning

½ teaspoon cayenne pepper (optional)

8 ounces cream cheese

1 cup heavy cream

PREP
5 minutes

SAUTÉ
10 minutes

PRESSURE COOK
5 minutes on High

RELEASE
Quick

TOTAL
30 minutes

- GLUTEN-FREE
- NUT-FREE

PER SERVING
Calories: 355; Total fat: 27g; Total carbs: 12g; Net carbs: 8g; Fiber: 4g; Sugar: 7g; Protein: 18g

MACROS
67% fat
13% carbs
20% protein

1. Select the pressure cooker's Sauté or Browning feature and adjust the heat to medium. Put the bacon in and sauté for 6 to 8 minutes, or until crisp. Using a slotted spoon, remove the bacon and transfer to a paper towel–lined plate to drain.
2. Add the garlic, onion, and celery to the bacon fat left in the cooker and sauté for 3 to 4 minutes.
3. Stir in the cauliflower, clams, clam juice, broth, thyme, 1 teaspoon of salt, ½ teaspoon of pepper, and the cayenne (if using) until well mixed.

4. Lock the lid into place and set the steam release knob to the sealed position. Set the pressure level to High and the time to 5 minutes. After cooking, quick release the pressure. Unlock and remove the lid.
5. Add the cream cheese, heavy cream, and cooked bacon. Stir until the cream cheese is melted. Season with more salt and pepper.
6. Divide the chowder among bowls and serve.

COOKING TIP: To thicken the soup, add 1 to 2 tablespoons of beef gelatin mixed with a few tablespoons of cool water or ½ teaspoon of xanthan gum after adding the cream, cream cheese, and bacon in step 5.

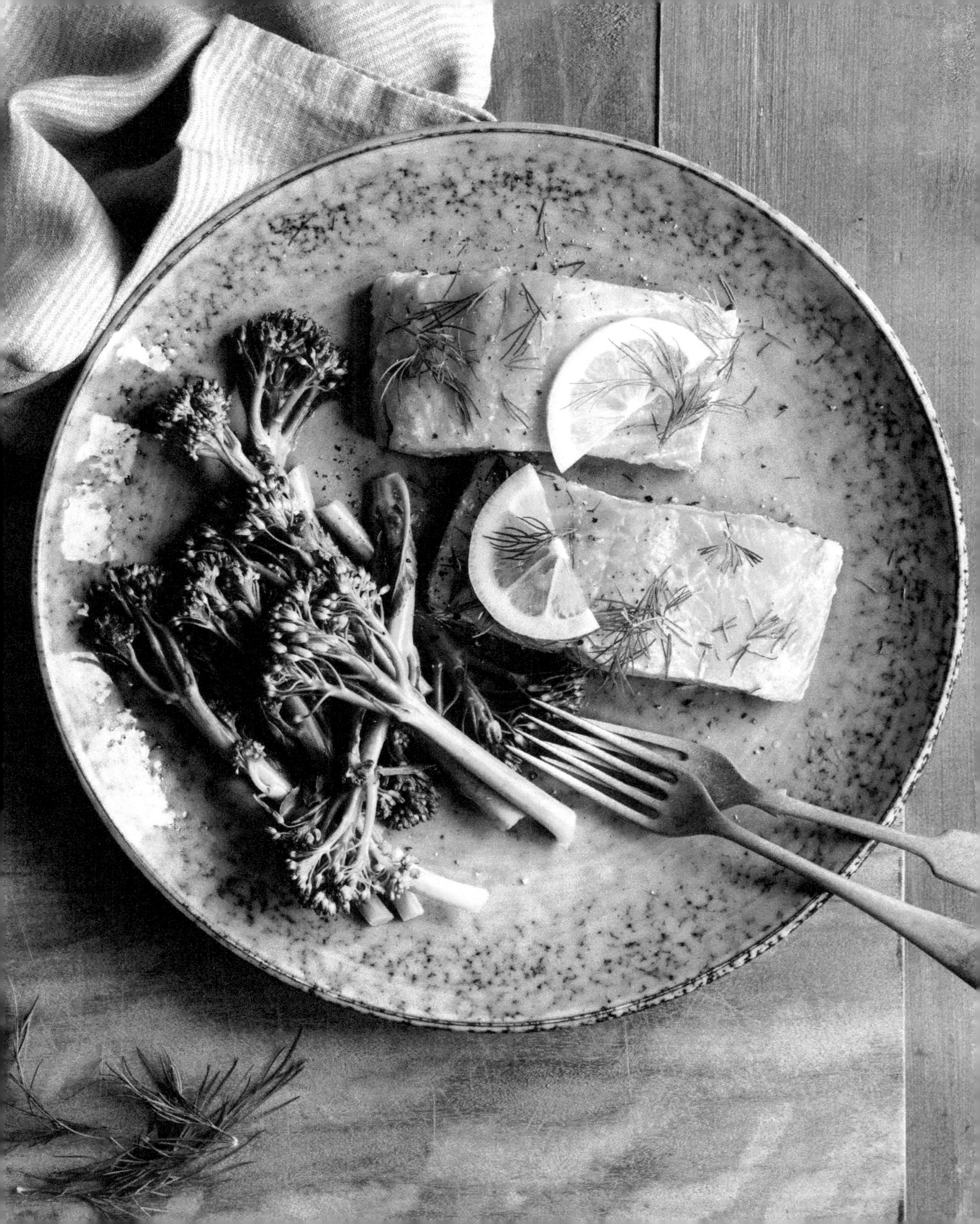

Chapter Six

Fish and Shellfish

(left) Simple Salmon and Broccolini

Coconut Fish Curry

This curry is very versatile. You can choose from a variety of fish, like halibut, tilapia, cod, or sea bass, and add additional vegetables, such as mushrooms and broccoli. Design the recipe to your liking or make it as written. Either way will be delicious. **SERVES 5**

3 tablespoons coconut oil

5 garlic cloves, minced

2 tablespoons minced fresh ginger

1 onion, sliced

1½ pounds mild white fish (I use sea bass), cut into 2-inch pieces

2 medium tomatoes, chopped

1 green bell pepper, chopped

1 (13.5-ounce) can full-fat coconut milk

2 tablespoons coconut aminos

1 tablespoon red curry paste

1 teaspoon fish sauce

1 teaspoon ground turmeric

1 teaspoon sea salt

½ teaspoon freshly ground black pepper

½ teaspoon paprika

½ teaspoon red pepper flakes

⅓ cup chopped fresh cilantro

Juice of 1 lime

PREP
2 minutes

SAUTÉ
5 minutes

PRESSURE COOK
2 to 3 minutes on High

RELEASE
Quick

TOTAL
20 minutes

- DAIRY-FREE
- GLUTEN-FREE
- NUT-FREE

PER SERVING
Calories: 362; Total fat: 22g; Total carbs: 13g; Net carbs: 11g; Fiber: 2g; Sugar: 9g; Protein: 30g

MACROS
54% fat
14% carbs
32% protein

1. Select the pressure cooker's Sauté or Browning feature and adjust the heat to medium. Heat the coconut oil in the cooker until shimmering. Add the garlic, ginger, and onion. Sauté for 3 to 5 minutes, or until the onion is translucent.
2. Add the fish, tomatoes, bell pepper, coconut milk, coconut aminos, red curry paste, fish sauce, turmeric, salt, pepper, paprika, and red pepper flakes and mix well.
3. Close and lock the lid and set the steam release knob to the sealed position. Set the pressure level to High and the time to 2 to 3 minutes, depending on the thickness of the fish fillets. After cooking, quick release the pressure. Unlock and remove the lid.
4. Garnish the fish with the cilantro, drizzle with the lime juice, and serve.

Snapper Veracruz

Red snapper Veracruz is a traditional dish from Mexico. This spicy, flavorful fish recipe is made with onions, tomatoes, jalapeños, and savory herbs. It is the perfect quick dinner entrée. **SERVES 4**

4 snapper fillets, about 5 ounces each

Kosher salt

Freshly ground black pepper

5 tablespoons extra-virgin olive oil, divided

½ small onion, sliced (about ½ cup)

2 large garlic cloves, minced

1 small jalapeño pepper, seeded and minced (about 1 tablespoon)

1 (14.5-ounce) can diced tomatoes, drained

¼ cup sliced green olives

1 bay leaf

½ teaspoon dried oregano

2 tablespoons chopped fresh parsley, divided

3 tablespoons capers, divided

PREP
10 minutes

PRESSURE COOK
5 minutes on High, plus 1 minute on High

RELEASE
Quick; Natural for 2 minutes, then Quick

TOTAL
30 minutes

- DAIRY-FREE
- GLUTEN-FREE
- NUT-FREE

PER SERVING (1 FILLET)
Calories: 343; Total fat: 20g; Total carbs: 7g; Net carbs: 2g; Fiber: 5g; Sugar: 3g; Protein: 30g

MACROS
55% fat
9% carbs
36% protein

1. On a plate, season the snapper fillets with salt and pepper, then put them in the refrigerator while you make the sauce.
2. Select the pressure cooker's Sauté or Browning feature and adjust the heat to high. Heat 4 tablespoons of olive oil in the cooker until shimmering. Add the onion and sprinkle with a pinch or two of salt. Cook, stirring, for about 5 minutes, or until the onion begins to brown. Add the garlic and jalapeño and cook for 1 to 2 minutes, or until the garlic is fragrant and the onion is mostly browned.
3. Add the tomatoes, olives, bay leaf, oregano, 1 tablespoon of parsley, and 1½ tablespoons of capers and mix well.

4. Lock the lid into place and set the steam release knob to the sealed position. Set the pressure level to High and the time to 5 minutes. After cooking, quick release the pressure. Unlock and remove the lid.

5. Remove the snapper from the refrigerator and place the fillets on top of the sauce. Lock the lid into place and set the steam release knob to the sealed position. Set the pressure level to High and the time to 1 minute. After cooking, let the pressure release naturally for 2 minutes, then quick release any remaining pressure. Unlock and remove the lid.

6. Check the fish with a fork to make sure it's cooked in the center. If not, put the lid back on the pressure cooker but do not lock it, and let the fish cook for 1 to 2 more minutes (the residual heat and steam will finish cooking it).

7. To serve, place the snapper fillets on a serving platter and spoon the sauce over top. Sprinkle with the remaining 1 tablespoon of parsley, 1½ tablespoons of capers, and 1 tablespoon of olive oil.

Simple Salmon and Broccolini

I make this recipe one or two times a week because it has high nutrient content, simple ingredients, and is done in under 30 minutes. It can be made from either fresh or frozen salmon. If using fresh, cut down the initial cook time on High to 1 to 2 minutes. **SERVES 4**

4 garlic cloves, minced

2 teaspoons chopped fresh dill

4 (4- to 6-ounce) fillets frozen wild-caught Alaskan salmon

Sea salt

Freshly ground black pepper

¼ cup unsalted grass-fed butter, plus 2 tablespoons melted

8 ounces broccolini

1 tablespoon onion powder

1. Rub the garlic and dill evenly on the salmon. Season with salt and pepper. Pour 1 cup of water into the pressure cooker and place the trivet inside. Arrange the salmon on the trivet. Place 1 tablespoon of butter on each of the salmon fillets.
2. Close and lock the lid and set the steam release knob to the sealed position. Set the pressure level to High and the time to 3 minutes. After cooking, quick release the pressure. Unlock and remove the lid.
3. Arrange the broccolini evenly on top of the salmon. Season with the onion powder, salt, and pepper. Lock the lid into place and set the steam release knob to the sealed position. Set the pressure level to Low and the time to 0 minutes.
4. After cooking, quick release the pressure and remove the broccolini and salmon from the pressure cooker. Serve with the remaining 2 tablespoons of melted butter.

PREP
2 minutes

PRESSURE COOK
3 minutes on High, plus 0 minutes on Low

RELEASE
Quick

TOTAL
15 minutes

- GLUTEN-FREE
- NUT-FREE

PER SERVING (1 FILLET)
Calories: 223; Total fat: 17g; Total carbs: 3g; Net carbs: 2g; Fiber: 1g; Sugar: 1g; Protein: 15g

MACROS
68% fat
4% carbs
28% protein

INGREDIENT TIP: Broccolini is a cross between broccoli and Chinese broccoli. It grows in slender, individual stalks and has a sweet, earthy taste. Regular broccoli can be substituted in this recipe if you cannot find broccolini.

Herb and Lemon Salmon

Fish and seafood are two of my favorites foods and have become only more delicious since I have started cooking them in a pressure cooker. Loaded with garlic, lemon, and herbs, this salmon is packed with flavor and has an amazing melt-in-your-mouth texture that I have not been able to achieve with other cooking methods. **SERVES 4**

¾ cup Avocado Oil Mayonnaise (page 21) or store-bought olive oil or avocado oil mayonnaise

3 tablespoons chopped fresh parsley, divided

1 tablespoon minced garlic

1 tablespoon freshly squeezed lemon juice

1 tablespoon finely grated lemon zest

2 teaspoons sea salt

1 pound wild-caught Alaskan salmon fillet, cut into four pieces

1. In a small bowl, combine the mayonnaise, 2 tablespoons of parsley, the garlic, lemon juice, lemon zest, and salt. Place each piece of salmon on a piece of aluminum foil, skin-side down. Spread the mayonnaise mixture evenly over the salmon and wrap each packet to seal.
2. Pour 1 cup of water into the pressure cooker and place the trivet inside. Arrange the foil packets on the trivet.
3. Lock the lid into place and set the steam release knob to the sealed position. Set the pressure level to High and the time to 3 minutes. After cooking, quick release the pressure.
4. Unlock and remove the lid. Remove the salmon packets from the pressure cooker.
5. Unwrap the salmon and sprinkle evenly with the remaining 1 tablespoon of parsley. Serve immediately.

PREP
7 minutes

PRESSURE COOK
3 minutes on High

RELEASE
Quick

TOTAL
20 minutes

- DAIRY-FREE
- GLUTEN-FREE
- NUT-FREE

PER SERVING (1 FILLET)
Calories: 302; Total fat: 19g; Total carbs: 7g; Net carbs: 4g; Fiber: 3g; Sugar: 0g; Protein: 23g

MACROS
60% fat
9% carbs
31% protein

COOKING TIP: The cook time will vary depending on the size and thickness of your salmon fillets. Three minutes is the perfect amount of time for fillets that are about 1 inch thick.

Shrimp Scampi

When the large shrimp boats come to dock near my house, I buy several pounds of fresh shrimp at a time. I clean them and freeze them in one-pound portions. My Instant Pot turns each portion of frozen shrimp into a delectable and fat-filled meal in under 30 minutes. **SERVES 4**

4 tablespoons unsalted grass-fed butter

4 tablespoons minced garlic

3 shallots, minced

½ cup dry white wine

1 pound frozen shrimp, peeled and deveined

Juice of 1 lemon

1 teaspoon sea salt

1 teaspoon freshly ground black pepper

1 teaspoon finely grated lemon zest

½ cup grated Parmesan cheese

3 cups Zucchini Noodles (page 29)

2 tablespoons chopped fresh parsley

1. Select the pressure cooker's Sauté or Browning feature, adjust the heat to high, and melt the butter in the cooker until it foams. Add the garlic and shallots and sauté for about 2 minutes, or until browned. Add the white wine and cook for 1 to 2 minutes, or until the alcohol burns off.
2. Add the frozen shrimp, lemon juice, salt, and pepper and stir to combine. Lock the lid into place and set the steam release knob to the sealed position. Set the pressure level to High and the time to 1 minute. After cooking, quick release the pressure. Unlock and remove the lid.
3. Select the pressure cooker's Sauté or Browning feature again and adjust the heat to high. Add the lemon zest and Parmesan cheese to the shrimp. Mix well and serve immediately over the zucchini noodles, garnished with the chopped parsley.

PREP
5 minutes

SAUTÉ
4 minutes

PRESSURE COOK
1 minute on High

RELEASE
Quick

TOTAL
20 minutes

- GLUTEN-FREE
- NUT-FREE

PER SERVING
Calories: 417; Total fat: 26g; Total carbs: 10g; Net carbs: 9g; Fiber: 1g; Sugar: 2g; Protein: 35g

MACROS
56% fat
10% carbs
34% protein

COOKING TIP: If you're making this recipe with fresh shrimp, set the timer to 0. Shrimp cooks very fast in a pressure cooker, and you don't want it to overcook and be rubbery.

Mussels with Garlic and Wine

Garlic, wine, and butter pair perfectly with mussels. This simple preparation enhances the flavor of the shellfish without completely overpowering the amazing taste of fresh seafood. **SERVES 4**

1 tablespoon avocado oil

1 shallot, sliced

Sea salt

Freshly ground black pepper

6 garlic cloves, minced

3 tablespoons unsalted grass-fed butter, divided

1 cup dry white wine

1 tablespoon dried thyme

1 tablespoon dried oregano

2 pounds mussels in shells, rinsed and debearded

¼ cup chopped fresh parsley

1. Select the pressure cooker's Sauté or Browning feature and adjust the heat to high. Heat the avocado oil in the cooker until shimmering, then add the shallot and season with salt and pepper. Sauté for about 5 minutes, until the shallot is starting to brown. Add the garlic and 1 tablespoon of butter and sauté for 1 to 2 minutes. Add the wine, thyme, and oregano and simmer for an additional 2 minutes.
2. Add the mussels. Close and lock the lid and set the steam release knob to the sealed position. Set the pressure level to High and the time to 3 minutes. After cooking, quick release the pressure. Unlock and remove the lid. Using a slotted spoon, transfer the mussels to serving bowls, discarding any that have not opened.
3. In the pressure cooker pot, combine the remaining 2 tablespoons of butter and the parsley and stir until the butter is melted. Pour the sauce over the mussels and season with salt and pepper.

PREP
3 minutes

SAUTÉ
9 minutes

PRESSURE COOK
3 minutes on High

RELEASE
Quick

TOTAL
25 minutes

- GLUTEN-FREE
- NUT-FREE

PER SERVING
Calories: 261; Total fat: 15g; Total carbs: 8g; Net carbs: 7g; Fiber: 1g; Sugar: 1g; Protein: 14g

MACROS
60% fat
14% carbs
26% protein

INGREDIENT TIP: Most mussels you purchase will be farmed and clean. If you are harvesting them yourself or can purchase wild mussels, be sure to scrub and soak them before cooking.

Jambalaya

This low-carb take on authentic jambalaya combines Cajun spices, seafood, and spicy sausage to satisfy all of my Southern-comfort-food cravings. I replaced the traditional rice with cauliflower to keep the consistency of the dish without all of the carbs. **SERVES 8**

- 1 large head cauliflower, separated into florets
- 4 tablespoons Ghee (page 18), divided
- 1 pound shrimp, peeled and deveined
- 1 pound boneless, skinless chicken thighs, chopped
- 1 pound andouille sausage, sliced
- 1 cup chopped onion
- 1 cup chopped green bell pepper
- 1 cup chopped celery
- 1 zucchini, sliced
- 1 tablespoon minced garlic
- 1 tablespoon dried thyme
- 1 tablespoon ground cumin
- 1 tablespoon smoked paprika
- 1 tablespoon onion powder
- ½ teaspoon cayenne pepper
- 1½ teaspoons sea salt
- 1 teaspoon Worcestershire sauce
- 1 cup dry white wine
- 1 (14.5-ounce) can diced tomatoes with their juices
- 2 tablespoons chopped fresh parsley
- 3 scallions, green parts only, sliced

PREP
5 minutes

SAUTÉ
8 minutes

PRESSURE COOK
2 minutes on High

RELEASE
Quick

TOTAL
25 minutes

- GLUTEN-FREE
- NUT-FREE

PER SERVING
Calories: 406; Total fat: 25g; Total carbs: 15g; Net carbs: 11g; Fiber: 4g; Sugar: 8g; Protein: 27g

MACROS
57% fat
15% carbs
28% protein

1. In a food processor, pulse the cauliflower until it is broken down into rice-size pieces. Remove the cauliflower from the food processor and set aside.
2. Select the pressure cooker's Sauté or Browning feature and adjust the heat to high. Melt 1 tablespoon of ghee in the cooker. Add the shrimp and sauté for a few minutes on each side, until the shrimp is opaque. Using a slotted spoon, transfer the shrimp to a plate and set aside.

3. Melt the remaining 3 tablespoons of ghee in the pressure cooker. Add the chicken, sausage, onion, bell pepper, celery, zucchini, and garlic and sauté for 3 to 4 minutes. Add the thyme, cumin, smoked paprika, onion powder, cayenne, salt, Worcestershire sauce, and white wine and let simmer for 1 to 2 minutes.
4. Add the tomatoes and their juices and stir until well mixed.
5. Lock the lid into place and set the steam release knob to the sealed position. Set the pressure level to High and the time to 2 minutes. After cooking, quick release the pressure. Unlock and remove the lid.
6. Select the pressure cooker's Sauté or Browning feature again and adjust the heat to high. Carefully stir in the riced cauliflower and cook, stirring, for 5 to 6 minutes, or until the cauliflower reaches the desired consistency. Add the shrimp back to the cooker, mix well, and serve the jambalaya in bowls, garnished with the chopped parsley and sliced scallion greens.

INGREDIENT TIP: For the best flavor, use fresh shrimp and andouille sausage. However, frozen shrimp can be used if necessary; cook it for just 1 minute on High pressure. If you can't find andouille sausage, kielbasa or chorizo are good substitute options.

Lobster Tail Salad

Living in Costa Rica means I have access to lots of delicious, fresh wild-caught seafood. Because of this, lobster has become one of my favorite dishes. Lobster meat has a sweet and delicate flavor, and is paired wonderfully with the lemon, shallots, and avocado in this recipe. Served over a bed of fresh greens and drizzled with olive oil, this meal is full of flavor and lots of healthy fats. **SERVES 4**

2 pounds lobster tails

1½ cups chicken stock

Juice from 1½ lemons, divided

½ cup Avocado Oil Mayonnaise (page 21) or store-bought avocado oil or olive oil mayonnaise

¼ cup chopped shallots

2 tablespoons finely chopped fresh tarragon

¼ teaspoon celery salt

¼ teaspoon freshly ground black pepper, plus more for seasoning

2 cups mixed greens or lettuce leaves

2 avocados, halved, pitted, peeled, and sliced

4 tablespoons extra-virgin olive oil

Sea salt

1. Using a chef's knife, cut the lobster tails in half lengthwise. Pour the chicken stock into the pressure cooker and place a trivet inside. Arrange the lobster tails on the trivet, shell-side down. Squeeze about one-third of the lemon juice over the lobster.
2. Lock the lid into place and set the steam release knob to the sealed position. Set the pressure level to High and the time to 4 minutes.
3. While the lobster tails are cooking, in a medium bowl, mix the mayonnaise, shallots, tarragon, celery salt, ¼ teaspoon of pepper, and the remaining lemon juice. Fill a large bowl with cold water.

PREP
5 minutes

PRESSURE COOK
4 minutes on High

RELEASE
Quick

TOTAL
20 minutes, plus 30 minutes to chill

- DAIRY-FREE
- GLUTEN-FREE
- NUT-FREE

PER SERVING
Calories: 583; Total fat: 38g; Total carbs: 10g; Net carbs: 4g; Fiber: 6g; Sugar: 1g; Protein: 46g

MACROS
61% fat
7% carbs
32% protein

4. After the lobster is done cooking, quick release the pressure. Unlock and remove the lid. Using tongs, carefully remove the lobster tails and transfer them to the bowl of cold water to stop the cooking.
5. After the lobster is cool enough to handle, remove the meat from the lobster shells and chop into small chunks. Add the lobster meat to the mayonnaise mixture and mix well. Transfer the bowl to the refrigerator for 30 minutes to chill.
6. Once cool, serve the lobster salad on a bed of mixed greens, topped with several slices of avocado and drizzled with the olive oil. Season with salt and pepper to taste.

INGREDIENT TIP: When following a high-fat diet or ketogenic diet, the types of fats you consume are very important. Avoid eating highly processed and refined oils found in conventional mayonnaise and instead opt to make your own or buy mayonnaise made from 100 percent avocado oil or olive oil.

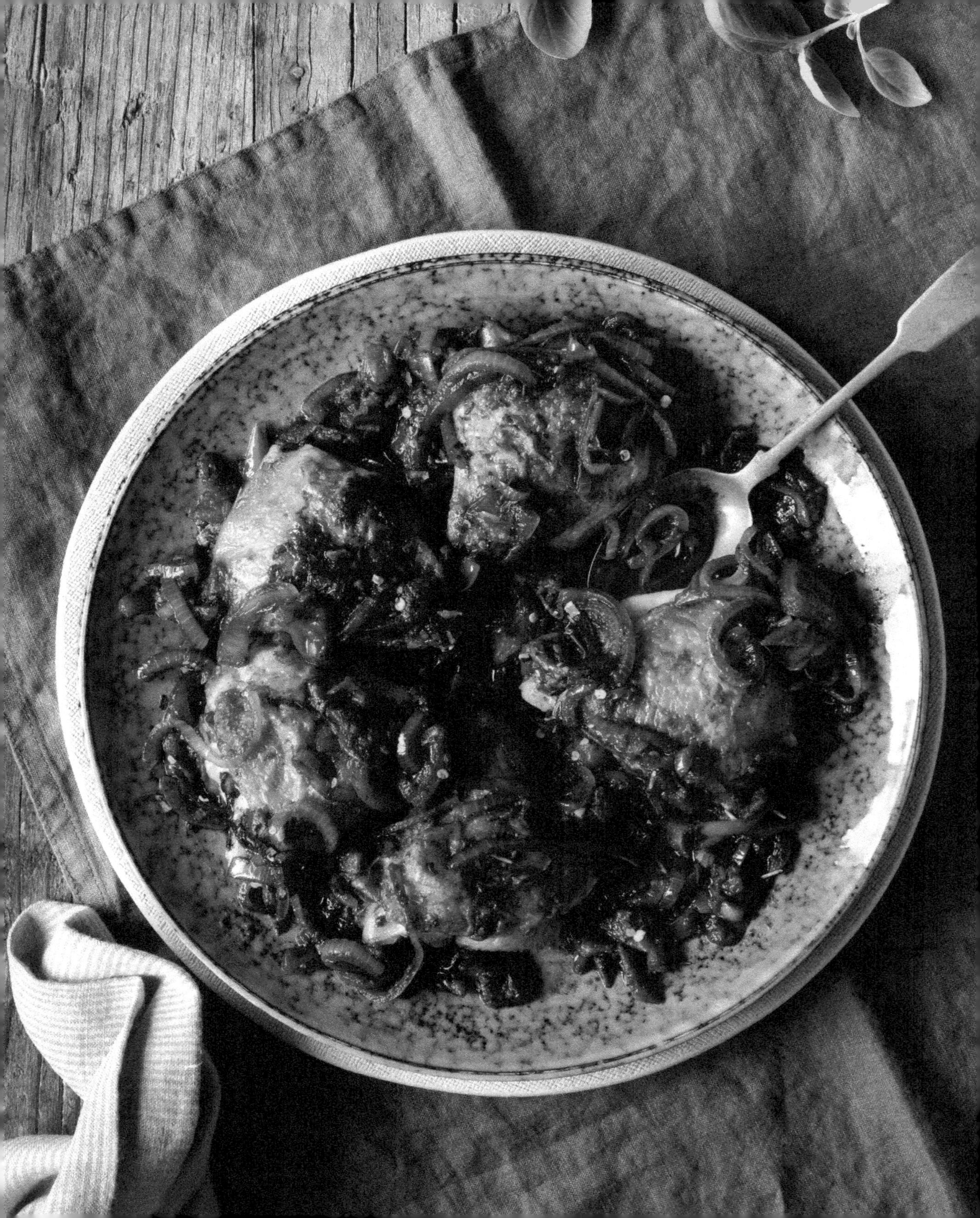

Chapter Seven

Poultry

(left) Balsamic Chicken Thighs

Barbecue Chicken Wings

This recipe is done in only 40 minutes and always a crowd favorite. Serve these savory wings with Avocado Ranch Dressing (page 23). **SERVES 6**

- 2 pounds split chicken wings
- ½ cup Sugar-Free Barbecue Sauce (page 26)
- ½ cup unsalted grass-fed butter, melted
- ½ teaspoon sea salt

1. Pour ¾ cup of water into the pressure cooker and place the trivet inside. Arrange the chicken wings on the trivet.
2. Lock the lid into place and set the steam release knob to the sealed position. Set the pressure level to High and the time to 5 minutes. After cooking, let the pressure release naturally.
3. While the pressure is releasing, in a small bowl, mix together the barbecue sauce, butter, and salt.
4. Preheat the oven to broil.
5. Once the pressure has finished releasing, unlock and remove the lid. Carefully remove the wings from the pressure cooker and transfer to a baking sheet. Brush the wings generously with the sauce and broil for 5 minutes. Remove the wings from the oven, flip them over to coat the opposite side with sauce, and broil for an additional 5 minutes, or until the wings reach the desired crispness.
6. Remove the wings from the oven and toss in the remaining sauce.

INGREDIENT SUBSTITUTION: Substitute the barbecue sauce for Frank's RedHot Wings sauce for buffalo style chicken wings.

PREP
5 minutes

PRESSURE COOK
5 minutes on High

RELEASE
Natural

BROIL
10 minutes

TOTAL
40 minutes

- GLUTEN-FREE
- NUT-FREE

PER SERVING
Calories: 474; Total fat: 40g; Total carbs: 2g; Net carbs: 2g; Fiber:0g; Sugar: 0g; Protein: 26g

MACROS
76% fat
2% carbs
22% protein

Creamy Salsa Verde Chicken

This is one of my favorite meal-prep dishes. It's quick, easy, and perfect on salads or in lettuce wraps. I have added spinach and avocado, so it can also easily be eaten by itself for a well-balanced high-fat and nutrient-dense meal. **SERVES 5**

- 1 tablespoon Ghee (page 18)
- 4 garlic cloves, minced
- 2 pounds boneless, skinless chicken thighs
- 1 teaspoon ground cumin
- 1 teaspoon sea salt
- ½ teaspoon freshly ground black pepper
- 1 jalapeño pepper, minced
- 1 (16-ounce) jar salsa verde
- 2 cups chopped spinach
- ½ cup cream cheese
- 1 avocado, halved, pitted, peeled, and chopped
- ¼ cup chopped fresh cilantro

1. Select the pressure cooker's Sauté or Browning feature, adjust the heat to medium, and heat the ghee until shimmering. Add the garlic and sauté until fragrant, about 1 to 2 minutes.
2. Add the chicken thighs, cumin, salt, pepper, jalapeño, and salsa verde.
3. Lock the lid into place and set the steam release knob to the sealed position. Set the pressure level to High and the time to 10 minutes. After cooking, quick release the pressure. Unlock and remove the lid.
4. Transfer the chicken thighs to a medium bowl and, using two forks, shred the meat.
5. Add the chopped spinach, cream cheese, and avocado to the leftover juices in the pressure cooker and stir until the spinach begins to wilt. Add the shredded chicken and stir. Garnish with the chopped cilantro and serve.

PREP
5 minutes

SAUTÉ
3 minutes

PRESSURE COOK
10 minutes on High

RELEASE
Quick

TOTAL
28 minutes

- GLUTEN-FREE
- NUT-FREE

PER SERVING
Calories: 399; Total fat: 26.6g; Total carbs: 9g; Net carbs: 7g; Fiber: 2g; Sugar: 5g; Protein: 31g

MACROS
60% fat
8% carbs
32% protein

INGREDIENT SUBSTITUTION: Dairy-free like me? Substitute coconut cream for the cream cheese.

Chicken Buffalo Meatballs

These meatballs are the perfect appetizer for tailgating or when hosting a party. The spicy kick of the hot sauce pairs perfectly with my Avocado Ranch Dressing (page 23). This combination is finger-licking good. **SERVES 4**

1 pound ground chicken

1 large egg

½ cup almond flour

1¼ cups hot sauce without added sugars, such as Frank's RedHot, divided

1 teaspoon garlic powder

1 teaspoon onion powder

½ teaspoon sea salt

¼ teaspoon freshly ground black pepper

2 tablespoons unsalted grass-fed butter

2 scallions, green parts only, sliced

1 recipe Avocado Ranch Dressing (page 23)

PREP
5 minutes

SAUTÉ
8 minutes

PRESSURE COOK
5 minutes on High

RELEASE
Natural

TOTAL
43 minutes

● GLUTEN-FREE

PER SERVING
Calories: 420; Total fat: 33g; Total carbs: 10g; Net carbs: 6g; Fiber: 4g; Sugar: 3g; Protein: 25g

MACROS
67% fat
9% carbs
24% protein

1. In a large bowl, combine the ground chicken, egg, almond flour, ¼ cup of hot sauce, the garlic powder, onion powder, salt, and pepper. Mix until the ingredients are well combined.
2. Using a small ice cream scoop or your hands, scoop 1-inch balls out of the meat mixture.
3. Select the pressure cooker's Sauté or Browning feature, adjust the heat to high, and melt the butter until shimmering. Add the meatballs to the pressure cooker in small batches. Brown evenly on all sides, 1 to 2 minutes per batch. Repeat until all of the meatballs are lightly browned, transferring them to a plate as they finish.

4. Once all of the meatballs are browned, scrape up any bits stuck to the bottom of the pan. Transfer the meatballs back to the pressure cooker and pour the remaining 1 cup of hot sauce over them.
5. Lock the lid into place and set the steam release knob to the sealed position. Set the pressure level to High and the time to 5 minutes. After cooking, let the pressure release naturally. Unlock and remove the lid. Transfer the meatballs to a platter and serve topped with the sliced scallion greens, with the ranch dressing for dipping.

Whole Chicken

Before owning a pressure cooker, I would buy a rotisserie chicken at the grocery store on a weekly basis. Cooking a whole chicken at home took more time and effort than I wanted to invest. However, using a pressure cooker makes cooking a faux-tisserie chicken so simple. The best part is that I get to control all the ingredients: nothing artificial, and no unwanted oils or added sugars. Just chicken, avocado oil, garlic, and spices make this juicy meal 100 percent clean.

SERVES 4

- 1 (3- to 4-pound) whole chicken
- ½ onion, cut into quarters
- 6 garlic cloves, crushed
- 1 lemon, halved
- 4 teaspoons sea salt
- 2 teaspoons paprika
- 1 teaspoon dried thyme
- 1 teaspoon freshly ground black pepper
- 1 teaspoon garlic powder
- ½ teaspoon cayenne pepper
- 2 tablespoons avocado oil, divided
- ½ cup chicken broth or water

PREP
10 minutes

SAUTÉ
8 minutes

PRESSURE COOK
24 to 28 minutes on High

RELEASE
Natural

TOTAL
1 hour 10 minutes

- DAIRY-FREE
- GLUTEN-FREE
- NUT-FREE

PER SERVING
Calories: 295; Total fat: 23g; Total carbs: 4g; Net carbs: 3g; Fiber: 1g; Sugar: 1g; Protein: 18g

MACROS
70% fat
5% carbs
25% protein

1. Remove the giblets from the chicken. Place the onion quarters, garlic, and lemon halves inside the cavity of the chicken. Use butcher's twine to tie the legs closed.
2. In a small bowl, mix together the salt, paprika, thyme, black pepper, garlic powder, and cayenne pepper. Rub the chicken with 1 tablespoon of avocado oil and then the spice mixture.
3. Select the pressure cooker's Sauté or Browning feature and adjust the heat to medium. Pour in the remaining 1 tablespoon of avocado oil and heat until shimmering. Place the chicken in the cooker and brown for about 4 minutes. Carefully flip and brown on the other side for 3 to 4 minutes.

4. Remove the chicken from the pressure cooker briefly in order to place the trivet inside, then place the chicken breast-side up on the trivet. Pour in the broth. Lock the lid into place and set the steam release knob to the sealed position. Set the pressure level to High and the time to 24 to 28 minutes (cooking time will vary depending on the size of your chicken; set the time for 8 minutes per pound).
5. After cooking, let the pressure release naturally. Unlock and remove the lid.
6. Remove the chicken from the pressure cooker and let rest for 5 to 10 minutes before serving.

LEFTOVER TIP: Save the carcass to make Bone Broth (page 19).

Chicken Cacciatore

This keto variation of the classic Italian dish can be made easily using a pressure cooker. The result is fall-off-the-bone chicken in a rich hearty sauce. I prefer my sauce to be thicker, so I sauté the sauce after the pressure cooking is complete, but if you are short on time, you can skip this step. **SERVES 6**

1½ pounds bone-in, skin-on chicken thighs

1 teaspoon sea salt, plus more for seasoning

¼ teaspoon freshly ground black pepper, plus more for seasoning

3 tablespoons Ghee (page 18)

1 onion, diced

5 garlic cloves, minced

1 red bell pepper, diced

1 (14.5-ounce) can diced tomatoes with their juices

½ cup dry white wine

1 teaspoon dried oregano

1 teaspoon onion powder

1 teaspoon dried thyme

1 teaspoon dried rosemary

¼ to ½ teaspoon red pepper flakes

½ cup pitted black olives

½ cup chopped fresh basil

½ cup grated Parmesan cheese

PREP
10 minutes

SAUTÉ
9 minutes

PRESSURE COOK
10 minutes on High

RELEASE
Quick

TOTAL
39 minutes

- GLUTEN-FREE
- NUT-FREE

PER SERVING
Calories: 419; Total fat: 30g; Total carbs: 10g; Net carbs: 7g; Fiber: 3g; Sugar: 6g; Protein: 22g

MACROS
68% fat
10% carbs
22% protein

1. Season the chicken on both sides with 1 teaspoon of salt and ¼ teaspoon of pepper. Select the pressure cooker's Sauté or Browning feature and adjust the heat to medium. Melt the ghee in the cooker until shimmering. Add the chicken thighs, skin-side down, and cook for 4 to 5 minutes, or until golden brown. Flip and cook for 1 to 2 minutes on the other side. Transfer the chicken thighs to a plate and set aside.
2. Put the onion, garlic, and bell pepper in the pressure cooker and sauté, stirring, for 1 to 2 minutes. Add the tomatoes and their juices, the wine, oregano, onion powder, thyme, rosemary, and red pepper flakes. Season with salt and pepper. Using a wooden spoon, stir well, scraping up any brown bits stuck to the bottom. Return the chicken thighs to the pressure cooker.

3. Lock the lid into place and set the steam release knob to the sealed position. Set the pressure level to High and the time to 10 minutes. After cooking, quick release the pressure. Unlock and remove the lid. Transfer the chicken thighs to a plate and set aside.
4. Select the pressure cooker's Sauté or Browning feature again and bring the sauce to a simmer. Add the olives and basil and simmer until the sauce is reduced to your desired consistency.
5. Return the chicken thighs to the pressure cooker and top with the Parmesan cheese. Season with salt and pepper and serve.

PAIRING TIP: This dish pairs perfectly with Spaghetti Squash (page 32) or Zucchini Noodles (page 29). Pairing with either of these sides would change the macros as follows: 72% fat, 9% carbs, 19% protein.

Cashew Chicken

Cashew chicken is a Chinese-American dish that is typically made with brown sugar and soy sauce. I have omitted the brown sugar and replaced the soy sauce with coconut aminos for a healthy variation of the dish. Instead of replacing the brown sugar with another keto-friendly sweetener, I eliminated it completely. Although sugar substitutes such as erythritol and stevia are keto-friendly, they should still be consumed in limited quantities. Just because something won't kick you out of ketosis doesn't mean it is good for you. **SERVES 4**

2 tablespoons coconut oil

1½ pounds boneless, skinless chicken thighs, cut into 1-inch pieces

½ cup coconut aminos

2 tablespoons apple cider vinegar

2 tablespoons fish sauce

2 garlic cloves, minced

1 tablespoon minced peeled fresh ginger

¼ teaspoon red pepper flakes

1 green bell pepper, diced

4 cups chopped broccoli florets

1 to 2 tablespoons grass-fed beef gelatin or ¼ to 1 teaspoon xanthan gum

1 cup toasted cashews

Sea salt

Freshly ground black pepper

2 tablespoons sesame seeds, for garnish

Sliced scallion greens, for garnish

1 tablespoon sesame oil, for garnish

PREP
5 minutes

SAUTÉ
2 minutes

PRESSURE COOK
5 minutes on High, plus 0 minutes on High

RELEASE
Quick

TOTAL
25 minutes

- DAIRY-FREE
- GLUTEN-FREE

PER SERVING
Calories: 419; Total fat: 25g; Total carbs: 15g; Net carbs: 12g; Fiber:3g; Sugar: 6g; Protein: 33g

MACROS
54% fat
14% carbs
32% protein

1. Select the pressure cooker's Sauté or Browning feature, adjust the heat to high, and heat the coconut oil until shimmering. Add the chicken and lightly brown for 1 to 2 minutes.
2. While the chicken is cooking, in a small bowl, whisk together the coconut aminos, apple cider vinegar, fish sauce, garlic, ginger, and red pepper flakes. Once the chicken is slightly browned, pour the sauce over chicken.

3. Lock the lid into place and set the steam release knob to the sealed position. Set the pressure level to High and the time to 5 minutes. After cooking, quick release the pressure. Unlock and remove the lid.
4. Stir in the bell pepper and broccoli. Lock the lid into place again and set the steam release knob to the sealed position and the time to 0 minutes. After cooking, quick release the pressure. Unlock and remove the lid.
5. In a small bowl, mix 1 tablespoon of gelatin into 4 to 5 tablespoons of cold water and let sit for 1 minute. Add half of the gelatin mixture to the chicken and mix until dissolved. Continue to add gelatin until the sauce reaches your desired consistency (the gelatin will continue to thicken as it cools). Repeat this process with additional gelatin and water if needed. Stir for 1 to 2 minutes, or until the sauce thickens.
6. Add the cashews and mix thoroughly. Season with salt and pepper. Serve garnished with the sesame seeds and sliced scallion greens and drizzled with sesame oil.

COOKING TIP: While I have eliminated the sugar in this recipe, if you are craving that sweet-and-sour taste, you can add a little stevia or your preferred sugar substitute to the sauce.

Butter Chicken

These tender chicken thighs are full of my favorite Indian spices and rich cream. This take on a restaurant favorite is ready in just over 30 minutes.
SERVES 6

- 5 tablespoons unsalted grass-fed butter
- 2 tablespoons minced peeled fresh ginger
- 6 garlic cloves, minced
- 1 (14.5-ounce) can diced tomatoes with their juices
- 2 teaspoons ground cumin
- 1 tablespoon garam masala
- 1 tablespoon ground coriander
- 1 tablespoon smoked paprika
- 1 teaspoon ground turmeric
- ½ teaspoon cayenne pepper
- 1 teaspoon sea salt
- 2 pounds boneless, skinless chicken thighs, cut into 2-inch cubes
- 1 cup full-fat coconut cream or heavy cream
- 1 tablespoon grass-fed beef gelatin or ¼ teaspoon xanthan gum (optional)
- ¼ cup chopped fresh cilantro

PREP
5 minutes

SAUTÉ
5 minutes

PRESSURE COOK
3 minutes on High

RELEASE
Natural for 10 minutes, then Quick

TOTAL
33 minutes

- GLUTEN-FREE
- NUT-FREE

PER SERVING
Calories: 409; Total fat: 27g; Total carbs: 7g; Net carbs: 5g; Fiber: 2g; Sugar: 2g; Protein: 32g

MACROS
61% fat
7% carbs
32% protein

1. Select the pressure cooker's Sauté or Browning feature and adjust the heat to medium. Melt the butter in the cooker until foaming. Add the ginger and garlic and sauté until aromatic.
2. Add the diced tomatoes and their juices, the cumin, garam masala, coriander, smoked paprika, turmeric, cayenne, and salt. Gently stir and cook for 3 to 5 minutes. Add the chicken and mix until it is fully coated in the sauce.
3. Lock the lid into place and set the steam release knob to the sealed position. Set the pressure level to High and the time to 3 minutes. After cooking, let the pressure release naturally for 10 minutes, then quick release any remaining pressure. Unlock and remove the lid.

4. Using a slotted spoon, remove the chicken and set aside. Pour the sauce from the pressure cooker into a blender and finely purée.
5. Select the pressure cooker's Browning or Sauté feature again, pour the sauce back into the cooker, and add the chicken. Add the coconut cream and mix well.
6. In a small bowl, mix 1 tablespoon of gelatin (if using) into 4 to 5 tablespoons of cold water and let sit for 1 minute. Add one-quarter of the gelatin mixture to the butter chicken and mix until dissolved. Continue to add gelatin until the sauce reaches your desired consistency (the gelatin will continue to thicken as it cools). Garnish the butter chicken with the cilantro and serve.

Chicken Shawarma

One of my favorite restaurants of all time is a little Middle Eastern place in my hometown, and chicken shawarma is my go-to order. As you might have guessed, there are no Middle Eastern restaurants in Costa Rica, but this recipe makes up for that and more. Topped with a tahini-garlic sauce, this dish has some of my all-time favorite flavors. It also pairs wonderfully with the tzatziki sauce from the Pork Gyro Lettuce Wraps (page 142). **SERVES 6**

2 pounds boneless, skinless chicken thighs, cut into pieces

1 tablespoon avocado oil

½ cup full-fat plain Greek yogurt

½ teaspoon ground cumin

½ teaspoon smoked paprika

½ teaspoon red pepper flakes

1 teaspoon dried oregano

1 teaspoon ground cardamom

½ teaspoon ground cinnamon

½ teaspoon ground allspice

2½ teaspoons sea salt, divided

¼ cup freshly squeezed lemon juice, plus 2 tablespoons

4 garlic cloves, minced, plus 2 garlic cloves, peeled

½ cup tahini

3 tablespoons extra-virgin olive oil

2 teaspoons chopped fresh parsley

Freshly ground black pepper

3 cups baby spinach

½ cup crumbled feta cheese

PREP
5 minutes, plus 2 hours to marinate

SAUTÉ
4 minutes

PRESSURE COOK
6 minutes on High

RELEASE
Quick

TOTAL
2 hours 27 minutes

- GLUTEN-FREE
- NUT-FREE

PER SERVING
Calories: 482; Total fat: 37g; Total carbs: 8g; Net carbs: 4g; Fiber: 4g; Sugar: 3g; Protein: 33g

MACROS
67% fat
6% carbs
27% protein

1. Place the chicken in a resealable bag. Add the avocado oil, yogurt, cumin, smoked paprika, red pepper flakes, oregano, cardamom, cinnamon, allspice, 2 teaspoons of salt, ¼ cup of lemon juice, and the minced garlic. Seal the bag and shake to evenly distribute the spices over the chicken. Let marinate in the refrigerator for 2 hours.
2. Select the pressure cooker's Sauté or Browning feature and adjust the heat to medium. Transfer the chicken to the cooker and sear for 1 to 2 minutes on each side. Add the marinade and ½ cup of water.
3. Lock the lid into place and set the steam release knob to the sealed position. Set the pressure level to High and the time to 6 minutes.
4. While the chicken is cooking, in a food processor, combine the tahini, olive oil, the 2 whole peeled garlic cloves, the remaining 2 tablespoons of lemon juice, the parsley, and the remaining ½ teaspoon of salt. Season with pepper and process until smooth.
5. After cooking the chicken, quick release the pressure. Unlock and remove the lid. Serve the chicken on plates over a bed of fresh spinach, topped evenly with the garlic sauce and feta.

COOKING TIP: Want crispy chicken shawarma? After the chicken has cooked in the pressure cooker, heat 1 to 2 tablespoons of oil in a pan and sauté the chicken until it starts to get crispy on the edges.

Mole Chicken

Mole negro is a traditional Mexican dish that is very labor-intensive and uses some difficult-to-find ingredients. My recipe is far from the traditional mole, but it is still very delicious. It pairs wonderfully with Coconut-Lime Cauliflower Rice (page 30) and Dairy-Free Sour Cream (page 22). **SERVES 6**

3 tablespoons coconut oil

1 onion, minced

5 garlic cloves, minced

1 (14.5-ounce) can diced tomatoes with their juices

2 pounds boneless, skinless chicken thighs

1 red bell pepper, minced

⅓ cup creamy peanut butter

1½ tablespoons chili powder

3 tablespoons cocoa powder

1 teaspoon ground cumin

1 chipotle chile in adobo sauce, diced

1 teaspoon adobo sauce

1 teaspoon ground cinnamon

½ teaspoon ground cloves

6 to 8 drops liquid stevia or preferred powdered sugar substitute equivalent to 1 to 2 tablespoons sugar (optional)

2 avocados, halved, pitted, peeled, and diced

¼ cup fresh chopped cilantro

PREP
5 minutes

SAUTÉ
10 minutes

PRESSURE COOK
15 minutes on High

RELEASE
Quick

TOTAL
40 minutes

- DAIRY-FREE
- GLUTEN-FREE

PER SERVING
Calories: 451; Total fat: 29g; Total carbs: 18g; Net carbs: 10g; Fiber: 8g; Sugar: 8g; Protein: 35g

MACROS
55% fat
15% carbs
30% protein

1. Select the pressure cooker's Sauté or Browning feature, adjust the heat to medium, and heat the coconut oil until shimmering. Add the onion and garlic and sauté until fragrant, about 1 to 2 minutes. Stir in the diced tomatoes and their juices and ½ cup water, scraping up any browned bits stuck to the bottom of the pot. Add the chicken.
2. Lock the lid into place and set the steam release knob to the sealed position. Set the pressure level to High and the time to 15 minutes. After cooking, quick release the pressure. Unlock and remove the lid.
3. Transfer the chicken to a bowl or work surface and, using two forks, shred the meat and set aside.
4. Select the pressure cooker's Sauté or Browning feature again and add the bell pepper, peanut butter, chili powder, cocoa powder, cumin, chipotle chile, adobo sauce, cinnamon, and cloves. Sauté for 5 to 8 minutes, or until the sauce is reduced by about half.
5. Use an immersion blender or stand blender to blend until smooth. Add the stevia (if using).
6. Pour the sauce over the chicken and mix thoroughly. Serve garnished with the diced avocado and chopped cilantro.

Balsamic Chicken Thighs

This simple and quick dish yields fragrant and juicy chicken with a tangy-sweet balsamic and tomato reduction sauce. Broiling the chicken after it is pressure cooked makes it perfectly crisp. **SERVES 6**

1½ pounds bone-in, skin-on chicken thighs

1 teaspoon sea salt

¼ teaspoon freshly ground black pepper

3 tablespoons Ghee (page 18)

1 large yellow onion, sliced

4 garlic cloves, minced

2 tomatoes, chopped

½ cup Bone Broth (page 19) or chicken broth

½ cup balsamic vinegar

2 teaspoons ground cumin

¼ teaspoon red pepper flakes

½ teaspoon dried rosemary

½ teaspoon ground cloves

½ teaspoon ground fennel

1 teaspoon dried oregano

6 to 8 drops liquid stevia or preferred powdered sugar substitute equivalent to 1 to 2 tablespoons sugar

¼ cup chopped fresh basil

PREP
5 minutes

SAUTÉ
20 minutes

PRESSURE COOK
10 minutes on High

RELEASE
Quick

TOTAL
45 minutes

- GLUTEN-FREE
- NUT-FREE

PER SERVING
Calories: 521; Total fat: 40g; Total carbs: 8g; Net carbs: 7g; Fiber: 1g; Sugar: 5g; Protein: 35g

MACROS
68% fat
6% carbs
26% protein

1. Season the chicken with the salt and pepper.
2. Select the pressure cooker's Sauté or Browning feature, adjust the heat to high, and heat the ghee until shimmering. Add the chicken thighs, skin-side down, and brown for 4 to 5 minutes, or until golden brown, then flip the chicken and cook for 1 to 2 minutes, or until golden brown on the other side. Remove the chicken thighs and set aside. Add the onion, garlic, and tomatoes to the pressure cooker and sauté for 2 to 3 minutes.
3. Add the bone broth, balsamic vinegar, cumin, red pepper flakes, rosemary, cloves, fennel, oregano, and stevia. Stir until mixed thoroughly, then return the chicken to the pot.

4. Lock the lid into place and set the steam release knob to the sealed position. Set the pressure level to High and the time to 10 minutes. After cooking, quick release the pressure. Unlock and remove the lid.
5. Preheat the oven to broil. Line a baking sheet with parchment paper.
6. Carefully remove the chicken thighs from the pressure cooker and transfer to the prepared baking sheet. Broil the chicken for 3 to 5 minutes, or until the skin begins to crisp.
7. While the chicken is broiling, switch the pressure cooker back to the Sauté or Browning function and simmer the sauce for 8 to 10 minutes, until it is reduced by about half.
8. Transfer the chicken to a serving bowl, pour the sauce over it, and serve garnished with the basil.

Chicken Korma

Don't let the long list of ingredients scare you away from this delicious korma recipe. The almonds, coconut, tomato, and spices combine to make a flavorful curry sauce. I love to serve this dish with Coconut-Lime Cauliflower Rice (page 30) or over a bed of fresh spinach. **SERVES 6**

3 tablespoons coconut oil

1 large yellow onion, sliced

4 garlic cloves, minced

2 tablespoons minced peeled fresh ginger

3 large tomatoes, diced

1 (13.5-ounce) can unsweetened coconut milk

¼ to ½ teaspoon red pepper flakes

2 tablespoons garam masala, divided

2 teaspoons ground coriander

1 teaspoon ground cumin

½ teaspoon ground turmeric

1 teaspoon fennel seeds

1 teaspoon ground cinnamon

½ teaspoon ground cloves

½ teaspoon ground nutmeg

¼ teaspoon cayenne pepper

1 teaspoon sea salt

¼ teaspoon freshly ground black pepper

2 pounds frozen boneless, skinless chicken thighs

½ cup grated unsweetened coconut

½ cup almond flour

¼ cup chopped fresh cilantro

PREP
8 minutes

SAUTÉ
3 minutes

PRESSURE COOK
10 minutes on High

RELEASE
Quick

SIMMER
15 minutes

TOTAL
46 minutes

- DAIRY-FREE
- GLUTEN-FREE

PER SERVING
Calories: 465; Total fat: 39g; Total carbs: 12g; Net carbs: 9g; Fiber: 3g; Sugar: 5g; Protein: 23g

MACROS
73% fat
9% carbs
18% protein

1. Select the pressure cooker's Sauté or Browning feature, adjust the heat to medium, and heat the coconut oil until shimmering. Add the onion, garlic, and ginger and sauté for 2 to 3 minutes.
2. Add the tomatoes, coconut milk, red pepper flakes, 1 tablespoon of garam masala, the coriander, cumin, turmeric, fennel, cinnamon, cloves, nutmeg, cayenne pepper, salt, black pepper, frozen chicken thighs, and ½ cup water. Stir until mixed.

3. Lock the lid into place and set the steam release knob to the sealed position. Set the pressure level to High and the time to 10 minutes. After cooking, quick release the pressure. Unlock and remove the lid.
4. Using a slotted spoon, carefully remove the chicken, transfer to a plate, and shred the meat into bite-size pieces. Set aside.
5. Using an immersion blender, blend the sauce in the pressure cooker until smooth, or transfer the sauce to a blender and mix until smooth. If using a stand blender, transfer the sauce back to the pressure cooker.
6. Add the remaining 1 tablespoon of garam masala, the grated coconut, and almond flour to the sauce. Select the pressure cooker's Sauté or Browning feature and simmer the sauce for 15 minutes, or until it is reduced by half.
7. Transfer the chicken back to the pressure cooker and mix with the sauce. Serve with the chopped cilantro.

Creamy Artichoke Chicken

This was one of the first recipes I made with my Instant Pot. I wanted to create a dairy-free variation for one of my favorite chicken-artichoke dips. The coconut cream gives it the same creamy and rich flavor but without the negative side effects that eating dairy can cause. I love to pair this dish with Spaghetti Squash (page 32) or Zucchini Noodles (page 29). **SERVES 6**

- 3 tablespoons avocado oil
- 1 onion, chopped
- 5 garlic cloves, minced
- 2 pounds boneless, skinless chicken thighs
- ½ cup Bone Broth (page 19) or chicken broth
- 1 tablespoon freshly squeezed lemon juice
- 1 tablespoon onion powder
- ¼ to ½ teaspoon red pepper flakes
- 1 teaspoon sea salt
- ¼ teaspoon freshly ground black pepper
- 1 (14-ounce) can chopped artichoke hearts, drained
- 4 cups fresh spinach
- ½ cup chopped fresh basil
- 1 cup full-fat coconut cream
- ½ cup Avocado Oil Mayonnaise (page 21)
- 1 teaspoon finely grated lemon zest

PREP
8 minutes

SAUTÉ
3 minutes

PRESSURE COOK
13 minutes on High

RELEASE
Quick

TOTAL
31 minutes

- DAIRY-FREE
- GLUTEN-FREE
- NUT-FREE

PER SERVING
Calories: 504; Total fat: 35g; Total carbs: 12g; Net carbs: 9g; Fiber: 3g; Sugar: 3g; Protein: 35g

MACROS
62% fat
10% carbs
28% protein

1. Select the pressure cooker's Sauté or Browning feature, adjust the heat to medium, and heat the avocado oil until shimmering. Add the onion and garlic and sauté for 2 to 3 minutes, or until the onion is translucent.
2. Add the chicken, broth, lemon juice, onion powder, red pepper flakes, salt, and pepper.
3. Lock the lid into place and set the steam release knob to the sealed position. Set the pressure level to High and the time to 13 minutes. After cooking, quick release the pressure. Unlock and remove the lid.

4. Transfer the chicken to a medium bowl and, using two forks, shred the meat into small pieces. Set aside.
5. Select the pressure cooker's Sauté or Browning feature again and add the chopped artichoke hearts, spinach, basil, coconut cream, mayonnaise, and lemon zest. Mix the ingredients well and cook until the sauce begins to thicken. Transfer the chicken back to the pressure cooker and stir to heat through.

INGREDIENT SUBSTITUTION: If you eat dairy, substitute cream cheese for the coconut cream and top the chicken with shredded Parmesan for a wonderful variation on this dish.

Homemade Sliced Turkey and Gravy

Cooking turkey and gravy in my Instant Pot has made this keto-friendly Thanksgiving dinner meal a frequent occurrence instead of a once-a-year treat. Pair this recipe with Cauliflower Purée (page 54) and Cheesecake (page 158), and you have a festive, fat-filled feast. **SERVES 8**

- 1 tablespoon dried thyme
- 1 tablespoon dried sage
- 1 tablespoon crushed garlic
- 1 teaspoon ground marjoram
- 1 teaspoon sea salt
- ½ teaspoon freshly ground black pepper
- ½ teaspoon ground nutmeg
- 3½ pounds bone-in, skin-on turkey breast
- 3 cups Bone Broth (page 19) or chicken broth, divided
- 1 onion, quartered
- 1 celery stalk, chopped
- 1 to 2 tablespoons grass-fed beef gelatin or ¼ to ½ teaspoon xanthan gum
- 1 tablespoon Ghee (page 18)

1. In a small bowl, mix together the thyme, sage, garlic, marjoram, salt, pepper, and nutmeg. Rub the spice mixture all over the turkey breast.
2. Put 2 cups of bone broth, the onion, and celery in the pressure cooker and place the trivet inside. Place the turkey breast skin-side up on the trivet.
3. Lock the lid into place and set the steam release knob to the sealed position. Set the pressure level to High and the time to 20 minutes. After cooking, let the pressure release naturally. Unlock and remove the lid. Using a kitchen thermometer, check the internal temperature of the turkey. It should read no lower than 165°F. If the turkey is not at 165°, lock the lid into place again and cook for an additional 5 to 7 minutes.

PREP
10 minutes

PRESSURE COOK
20 minutes on High

RELEASE
Natural

SAUTÉ
20 minutes

TOTAL
1 hour 15 minutes

- GLUTEN-FREE
- NUT-FREE

PER SERVING
Calories: 733; Total fat: 59g; Total carbs: 2g; Net carbs: 3g; Fiber: 0g; Sugar: 1g; Protein: 46g

MACROS
73% fat
1% carbs
26% protein

4. Remove the turkey breast from the pressure cooker and transfer to a serving platter. Tent with foil to keep warm.

5. Using a metal strainer, separate the solids from the turkey drippings. Discard the solids and place the drippings back in the pressure cooker.

6. Select the pressure cooker's Sauté or Browning feature and adjust the heat to low. Pour in the remaining 1 cup of bone broth. Allow the drippings and broth to simmer for 20 minutes. Once the time is almost complete, add the thickener of your choice. If using beef gelatin, mix 1 tablespoon of gelatin into 4 to 5 tablespoons of cold water and let sit for 1 minute. Add to the gravy and mix until dissolved. Add the remaining tablespoon of gelatin mixed with an additional 4 to 5 tablespoons of water as needed to reach your desired consistency (the gelatin will thicken as it cools). If using xanthan gum, stir in ¼ teaspoon at a time until the gravy reaches your desired consistency.

7. Mix the ghee into the gravy and season with salt and pepper. Let cool slightly before serving.

8. Carve the turkey breast and served smothered in gravy.

COOKING TIP: Grass-fed beef gelatin is a wonderful, healthy substitute for flour or other thickening agents. Gelatin has been shown to improve gut health, protect joints, and improve the health of skin and hair. Be aware that gelatin will continue to thicken as it cools. Xanthan gum can also be used to thicken low-carb soups and sauces. A little goes a long way—always add to recipes in increments of just ¼ teaspoon at a time.

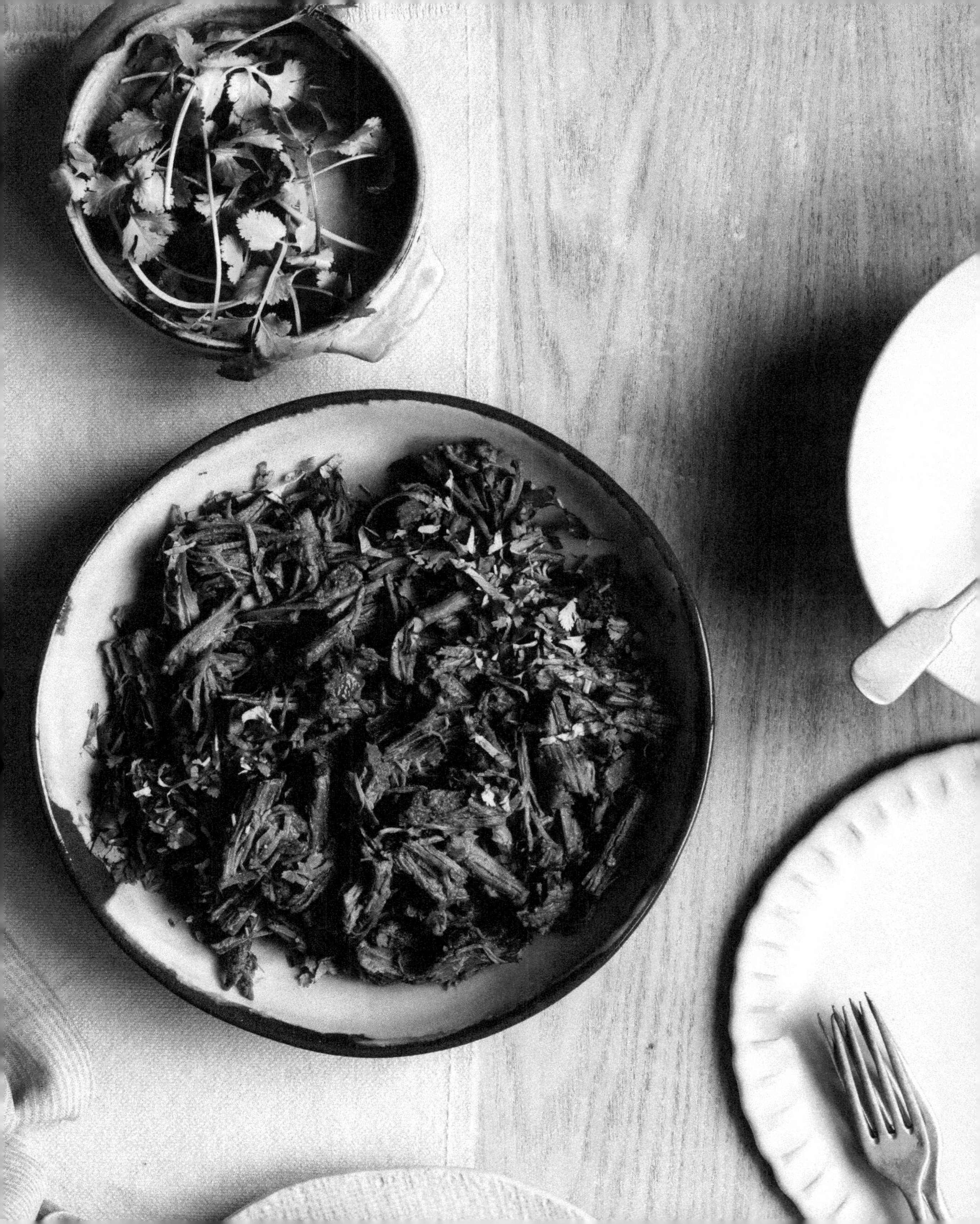

Chapter Eight

Beef and Pork

(left) Barbacoa Beef

Perfect Italian Meatballs

Spaghetti and meatballs were once my favorite comfort food. However, this recipe now easily takes its place. The sauce is packed full of spinach and pairs perfectly with Spaghetti Squash (page 32) or Zucchini Noodles (page 29) to deliver a delicious and guilt-free comfort food. This dish is loaded with Italian flavors and juicy texture to ensure that I never miss the spaghetti. **SERVES 7**

2 large eggs

1½ pounds grass-fed ground beef

½ cup almond flour

1 tablespoon nutritional yeast

½ cup minced onion

4 garlic cloves, crushed, divided

1 teaspoon dried oregano

1 teaspoon onion powder

1 teaspoon sea salt

½ teaspoon freshly ground black pepper

½ teaspoon red pepper flakes

2 tablespoons Ghee (page 18)

1 (24-ounce) can tomato sauce (no sugar added)

½ cup chopped fresh basil

3 cups chopped fresh spinach

2 tablespoons red wine

1 cup freshly grated Parmesan cheese

3 tablespoons extra-virgin olive oil

PREP
15 minutes

PRESSURE COOK
10 minutes on High

RELEASE
Quick

SAUTÉ
10 minutes

TOTAL
50 minutes

● GLUTEN-FREE

PER SERVING
Calories: 477; Total fat: 36g; Total carbs: 10g; Net carbs: 8g; Fiber: 2g; Sugar: 5g; Protein: 28g

MACROS
68% fat
8% carbs
24% protein

1. In a large bowl, beat the eggs. Add the beef, almond flour, nutritional yeast, onion, half of the crushed garlic, the oregano, onion powder, salt, black pepper, and red pepper flakes. Mix all the ingredients until just combined, then form into about 15 (1½- to 2-inch) meatballs.
2. Select the pressure cooker's Sauté or Browning feature, adjust the heat to medium, and melt the ghee until shimmering. Add the remaining crushed garlic and sauté until fragrant. Add the tomato sauce and 1 cup of water.

3. Let the sauce come to a simmer, then add the meatballs and basil.
4. Lock the lid into place and set the steam release knob to the sealed position. Set the pressure level to High and the time to 10 minutes. After cooking, quick release the pressure. Unlock and remove the lid.
5. Select the pressure cooker's Sauté or Browning feature again and mix in the spinach and red wine. Sauté until the spinach beings to wilt.
6. Serve the meatballs topped with the grated Parmesan cheese and drizzled with the olive oil.

COOKING TIP: For a thicker sauce, remove the meatballs with a slotted spoon after the pressure is released in step 4 and switch the pressure cooker back to Sauté or Browning. Let the sauce simmer for 8 to 10 minutes to reduce. After the sauce reaches the desired thickness, return the meatballs to the pressure cooker and continue with the recipe as written.

Taco Meat

This couldn't-be-easier taco meat goes straight from the freezer to the pressure cooker. It uses homemade taco seasoning instead of store-bought because of all the added sugars and starches found in those premade taco seasonings. Most of them also contain 15 to 20 grams of carbs per package. **SERVES 4**

- 1¼ pounds frozen grass-fed ground beef
- 2 tablespoons Ghee (page 18)
- 3 garlic cloves, minced
- ½ onion, minced
- 1 tablespoon ground cumin
- 2 teaspoons chili powder
- 1 tablespoon onion powder
- ¼ teaspoon cayenne pepper
- 2 teaspoons smoked paprika
- ½ teaspoon ground coriander
- ½ teaspoon ground cinnamon
- ½ teaspoon dried oregano
- ½ teaspoon sea salt
- ½ teaspoon freshly ground black pepper
- 4 cups mixed salad greens
- 2 cups Guacamole (page 27)
- 4 tablespoons Dairy-Free Sour Cream (page 22)

PREP
2 minutes

PRESSURE COOK
18 minutes on High

RELEASE
Quick

SAUTÉ
5 minutes

TOTAL
35 minutes

- GLUTEN-FREE
- NUT-FREE

PER SERVING
Calories: 582; Total fat: 52g; Total carbs: 23g; Net carbs: 10g; Fiber: 13g; Sugar: 3g; Protein: 39g

MACROS
65% fat
12% carbs
23% protein

1. Pour 1 cup of water into the pressure cooker and place the trivet inside. Place the frozen beef on the trivet.
2. Lock the lid into place and set the steam release knob to the sealed position. Set the pressure level to High and the time to 18 minutes. After cooking, quick release the pressure. Unlock and remove the lid.
3. Using tongs, remove the beef and set aside. It's fine if the beef is not cooked completely at this point, because it will continue to cook in the following steps. Pour off and reserve any accumulated liquids from the pressure cooker.

4. Select the pressure cooker's Sauté or Browning feature, adjust the heat to medium, and heat the ghee until shimmering. Add the garlic and onion and sauté until fragrant.
5. Return the beef to the pressure cooker and, using a wooden spoon, crumble into small pieces. Continue to sauté until cooked through. Add ¼ cup of the reserved cooking liquid along with the cumin, chili powder, onion powder, cayenne pepper, paprika, coriander, cinnamon, oregano, sea salt, and black pepper. Sauté until the liquid is mostly evaporated.
6. Serve the taco meat over the mixed greens, topped with the guacamole and sour cream.

INGREDIENT SUBSTITUTION: If you are not sensitive to dairy, feel free to use regular sour cream in this recipe instead of dairy-free sour cream.

Beef and Broccoli

This recipe uses one my favorite condiments, coconut aminos. Coconut aminos is my staple for Asian-inspired dishes because it is the perfect substitute for soy sauce, delivering that same salty-sweet flavor without any soy, gluten, or wheat. Coconut aminos brings this beef and broccoli dish to life. **SERVES 6**

1½ pounds grass-fed chuck roast, thinly sliced

½ teaspoon sea salt

Freshly ground black pepper

4 tablespoons coconut oil, divided

½ cup coconut aminos

½ cup Bone Broth (page 19) or beef stock

6 to 8 drops liquid stevia or preferred powdered sugar substitute equivalent to 1 to 2 tablespoons sugar (optional)

½ teaspoon red pepper flakes

1 tablespoon minced fresh ginger

2 shallots, minced

4 garlic cloves, minced

1 pound broccoli florets

1 to 2 tablespoons grass-fed beef gelatin or ¼ to ½ teaspoon xanthan gum (optional)

Sesame seeds, for garnish

Sliced scallion greens, for garnish

PREP
10 minutes

SAUTÉ
6 minutes

PRESSURE COOK
12 minutes on High

RELEASE
Quick

TOTAL
38 minutes

- DAIRY-FREE
- GLUTEN-FREE
- NUT-FREE

PER SERVING
Calories: 441; Total fat: 25g; Total carbs: 9g; Net carbs: 7g; Fiber: 2g; Sugar: 5g; Protein: 28g

MACROS
60% fat
9% carbs
31% protein

1. Season the beef with salt and pepper and rub with 2 tablespoons of coconut oil. Set aside. In a small bowl, combine the coconut aminos, bone broth, stevia (if using), red pepper flakes, and ginger.
2. Select the pressure cooker's Sauté or Browning feature, adjust the heat to medium, and heat the remaining 2 tablespoons of coconut oil until shimmering. Add the shallots and garlic and sauté for 1 to 2 minutes. Add the beef to the pot and sear for 1 to 2 minutes on each side, or until lightly browned. Pour the sauce mixture over the beef.

3. Lock the lid into place and set the steam release knob to the sealed position. Set the pressure level to High and the time to 12 minutes.
4. While the beef is cooking, place the broccoli in a microwave-safe bowl with ¼ cup water. Microwave for 2 to 3 minutes, or until the broccoli is tender.
5. After the beef has finished cooking, quick release the pressure. Unlock and remove the lid.
6. Select the pressure cooker's Sauté or Browning feature again and simmer the sauce until it begins to thicken. Mix in the gelatin or xanthan gum (if using). For the gelatin, mix 1 tablespoon into 4 to 5 tablespoons of cold water and let sit for 1 minute. Add half of the gelatin mixture to the sauce and mix until dissolved. Continue to add gelatin until it reaches the desired consistency (it will continue to thicken as it cools). Repeat this process with the remaining tablespoon of gelatin and additional water, if needed. For xanthan gum, a little goes a long way. Add ¼ teaspoon at a time to the beef and sauce, until thickened.
7. Stir the beef and sauce for 1 to 2 minutes, until the sauce thickens.
8. Add the broccoli and mix thoroughly. Garnish with sesame seeds and sliced scallion greens.

Beef Bourguignon

This recipe is inspired by the famous Julia Child's Beef Bourguignon. It is simplified by using the pressure cooker but still has the same rich, amazing flavor. I love to serve this dish over Basic Cauliflower Rice (page 30) or Spaghetti Squash (page 32). **SERVES 4**

- 10 thick bacon slices, chopped
- 1½ pounds grass-fed chuck roast, cut into 1-inch pieces
- 3 tablespoons unsalted grass-fed butter
- 6 garlic cloves, minced
- 2 carrots, sliced
- 1 cup sliced mushrooms
- 2 cups frozen pearl onions
- 2 tablespoons tomato paste
- 2 cups red wine
- ½ cup beef Bone Broth (page 19) or beef broth
- 1 teaspoon dried thyme
- 1 bay leaf
- 2 teaspoons sea salt
- ¼ teaspoon freshly ground black pepper
- 1 to 2 tablespoons grass-fed beef gelatin or ¼ to ½ teaspoon xanthan gum (optional)
- ¼ cup chopped fresh parsley

PREP
8 minutes

SAUTÉ
18 minutes

PRESSURE COOK
30 minutes on High

RELEASE
Quick

SIMMER
8 minutes

TOTAL
1 hour 6 minutes

- GLUTEN-FREE
- NUT-FREE

PER SERVING
Calories: 583; Total fat: 28g; Total carbs: 8g; Net carbs: 6g; Fiber: 2g; Sugar: 4g; Protein: 33g

MACROS
61% fat
8% carbs
31% protein

1. Select the pressure cooker's Sauté or Browning feature, adjust the heat to medium, and sauté the bacon until crisp. Transfer the bacon to paper towels to drain, leaving the rendered bacon fat in the cooker.
2. In small batches, add the beef and cook for 3 to 5 minutes, browning on all sides. Repeat until all the beef is browned. Set the browned beef aside.
3. Melt the butter in the pressure cooker until foaming. Add the garlic, carrots, and mushrooms and sauté for 2 to 3 minutes, stirring occasionally.
4. Add the beef, onions, tomato paste, wine, broth, thyme, bay leaf, salt, and pepper to the pot.

5. Lock the lid into place and set the steam release knob to the sealed position. Set the pressure level to High and the time to 30 minutes. After cooking, quick release the pressure. Unlock and remove the lid.
6. Return the pressure cooker to the Sauté or Browning setting. Simmer the sauce for 6 to 8 minutes, or until it is thickened and the alcohol cooks off.
7. If desired, mix 1 tablespoon of gelatin into 4 to 5 tablespoons of cold water and let sit for 1 minute. Add half of the gelatin mixture to the sauce and mix until dissolved. Continue to add gelatin until it reaches the desired consistency (the gelatin will continue to thicken as it cools). Repeat this process with additional gelatin and water if needed. For xanthan gum, add ¼ teaspoon at a time until thickened. Stir for an additional 1 to 2 minutes, until the sauce thickens.
8. Stir the bacon into the beef bourguignon and serve garnished with the parsley.

INGREDIENT TIP: To keep the carb count down, pick a dry red wine such as a Burgundy or Cabernet. Also pick a wine you enjoy drinking, because as the wine cooks down the flavors will come out.

Philly Cheesesteak

This keto variation on the classic Philadelphia cheesesteak is made from thinly sliced pieces of steak, peppers and onions, and melted cheese. Pair this gooey and delightful recipe with a side salad or green vegetable of your choice for a well-rounded, keto-friendly meal. **SERVES 6**

2 tablespoons unsalted grass-fed butter

2 large yellow onions, sliced

1 teaspoon sea salt, divided

4 garlic cloves, minced

3 green bell peppers, sliced

2 pounds grass-fed sirloin steak, thinly sliced

½ teaspoon freshly ground black pepper

1 tablespoon onion powder

1 tablespoon Worcestershire sauce

1 teaspoon dried oregano

½ cup Bone Broth (page 19) or beef broth

6 provolone cheese slices

1. Select the pressure cooker's Sauté or Browning feature, adjust the heat to medium, and heat the butter until foaming. Add the onions and ½ teaspoon of salt and sauté for 8 to 10 minutes, or until browned. Add the garlic and bell peppers and sauté for 2 to 3 minutes, or until the peppers soften. Remove the vegetables from the pressure cooker and set aside.
2. Add the sliced steak to the pressure cooker and season with the remaining ½ teaspoon of salt, the pepper, onion powder, Worcestershire sauce, and oregano. Pour in the broth.
3. Lock the lid into place and set the steam release knob to the sealed position. Set the pressure level to High and the time to 4 minutes. After cooking, quick release the pressure. Unlock and remove the lid.

PREP
5 minutes

SAUTÉ
13 minutes

PRESSURE COOK
4 minutes on High

RELEASE
Quick

BROIL
3 minutes

TOTAL
35 minutes

- GLUTEN-FREE
- NUT-FREE

PER SERVING
Calories: 566; Total fat: 39g; Total carbs: 12g; Net carbs: 8g; Fiber: 4g; Sugar: 5g; Protein: 40g

MACROS
62% fat
9% carbs
29% protein

4. Stir the onions and peppers into the steak until heated through.
5. Preheat the oven to broil. Line a baking sheet with parchment paper.
6. Using a slotted spoon, transfer the meat and vegetables to the prepared baking sheet and top with the cheese slices. Broil for 2 to 3 minutes, or until the cheese is melted.

PREP TIP: Freeze the beef for 30 minutes to make it easier to slice into superthin strips.

Barbacoa Beef

This is a fabulous meal-prep dish for serving large groups. You can set it and leave it and the result is melt-in-your-mouth, spicy beef. I love to serve this at a keto taco night with romaine lettuce (chopped or used as cups), diced tomatoes, sliced avocados, and sour cream or Dairy-Free Sour Cream (page 22).

SERVES 8

- 1 onion, minced
- 6 garlic cloves, minced
- 2 to 4 chipotle chiles in adobo sauce, minced
- ½ cup freshly squeezed lime juice
- 2 tablespoons apple cider vinegar
- 2 tablespoons ground cumin
- 1 tablespoon dried oregano
- ½ teaspoon ground cloves
- ½ cup Bone Broth (page 19) or beef broth
- 3 pounds grass-fed beef brisket, cut into 2- to 3-inch chucks
- 1 teaspoon sea salt
- ¼ teaspoon freshly ground black pepper
- 3 tablespoons avocado oil
- ¼ cup chopped fresh cilantro

PREP
5 minutes

SAUTÉ
13 minutes

PRESSURE COOK
60 minutes on High

RELEASE
Quick

TOTAL
1 hour 20 minutes

- DAIRY-FREE
- GLUTEN-FREE
- NUT-FREE

PER SERVING
Calories: 414; Total fat: 31g; Total carbs: 5g; Net carbs: 4g; Fiber: 1g; Sugar: 1g; Protein: 27g

MACROS
69% fat
5% carbs
26% protein

1. In a small bowl, whisk together the onion, garlic, chipotles, lime juice, apple cider vinegar, cumin, oregano, cloves, and broth. Set aside.
2. In a medium bowl, season the beef chunks with salt and pepper. Select the pressure cooker's Sauté or Browning feature, adjust the heat to medium, and heat the avocado oil until shimmering. Add the beef and turn every few minutes until browned on most sides, about 6 to 8 minutes total. Pour the sauce into the pressure cooker, scraping up any browned bits with a wooden spoon.

3. Lock the lid into place and set the steam release knob to the sealed position. Set the pressure level to High and the time to 60 minutes. After cooking, quick release the pressure. Unlock and remove the lid.
4. Using a slotted spoon, transfer the beef to a bowl and, using two forks, shred the meat. Transfer it back to the sauce. Serve the beef topped with the cilantro.

Italian Meatloaf

This is a wonderful keto variation on classic Italian meatloaf. I have used almond flour and eggs as the binding agents, and the meatloaf is topped with a wonderful fresh basil and tomato sauce. Serve this with a side of green veggies sautéed in butter for a perfect and well-rounded high-fat meal. **SERVES 8**

1½ pounds grass-fed ground beef

½ cup almond flour

½ cup grated Parmesan cheese

½ onion, minced

9 garlic cloves, minced, divided

⅓ cup tomato paste

2 tablespoons Worcestershire sauce

2 large eggs, whisked

1½ teaspoons dried oregano, divided

1 teaspoon onion powder

1½ teaspoons dried parsley, divided

½ teaspoon dried rosemary

1½ teaspoons sea salt, divided, plus more for seasoning

¼ teaspoon freshly ground black pepper, plus more for seasoning

2 tablespoons unsalted grass-fed butter

2 cups crushed tomatoes

1 bay leaf

½ cup chopped fresh basil

PREP
10 minutes

PRESSURE COOK
20 minutes on High

BROIL
5 minutes

RELEASE
Quick

TOTAL
45 minutes

● GLUTEN-FREE

PER SERVING
Calories: 515; Total fat: 33g; Total carbs: 12g; Net carbs: 9g; Fiber: 3g; Sugar: 5g; Protein: 42g

MACROS
58% fat
9% carbs
33% protein

1. In a large bowl, combine the ground beef, almond flour, Parmesan, onion, half of the minced garlic, the tomato paste, Worcestershire sauce, eggs, 1 teaspoon of oregano, the onion powder, 1 teaspoon of parsley, the rosemary, 1 teaspoon of salt, and the pepper. Mix with your hands until just combined.
2. Gently form the meat mixture into a loaf shape. Place the meatloaf on a double layer of aluminum foil. Wrap the foil around the sides of the meatloaf to create a foil pan, and ensure that the meatloaf and foil wrap can fit into the pressure cooker.

3. Pour 1 cup of water into the pressure cooker and place a trivet inside. Make a sling with aluminum foil by folding a long piece of foil into thirds. Use the sling to lower the meatloaf into the pressure cooker.
4. Lock the lid into place and set the steam release knob to the sealed position. Set the pressure level to High and the time to 20 minutes.
5. While the meatloaf is cooking, in a small saucepan, melt the butter over medium heat. Add the remaining minced garlic and sauté until fragrant. Add the crushed tomatoes, the remaining ½ teaspoon each of oregano, parsley, and salt, and the bay leaf and simmer for 15 minutes.
6. Remove the tomato sauce from the heat and add the basil. Taste and season with more salt and pepper, as desired. Set aside.
7. Preheat the oven to broil. Line a baking sheet with aluminum foil.
8. After the meatloaf is done cooking, quick release the pressure. Unlock and remove the lid, and use the foil sling to remove the meatloaf. Use a food thermometer to confirm that the meatloaf's internal temperature is at least 155°F. If it is not, return the meatloaf to the pressure cooker for 3 to 5 more minutes under High pressure and quick release the pressure after cooking.
9. Brush the tomato sauce over the top of the meatloaf and transfer to the prepared baking sheet. Broil on the top rack of the oven for 3 to 5 minutes, or until the top of the meatloaf begins to brown. Remove from the oven and serve with any remaining tomato sauce.

Pork Gyro Lettuce Wraps with Tzatziki

Greece is at the top of my bucket list of places I want to travel. I love the culture and the food! These Greek-inspired lettuce wraps have tender pork, soft onions, and fresh cucumber tzatziki sauce. They are paired perfectly with sliced olives and fresh feta cheese. **SERVES 8**

FOR THE PORK LETTUCE WRAPS

- 4 tablespoons Ghee (page 18), at room temperature, divided
- 2 tablespoons minced garlic
- 1 teaspoon dried marjoram
- 1 teaspoon dried rosemary
- 1 teaspoon sea salt
- ¼ teaspoon freshly ground black pepper
- 3 pounds boneless pork shoulder, cut into 1-inch cubes
- 1 onion, sliced
- ½ cup freshly squeezed lemon juice
- ¼ cup Bone Broth (page 19) or beef broth
- 16 romaine lettuce leaves
- ½ cup sliced Kalamata olives
- ½ cup crumbled feta cheese

FOR THE TZATZIKI

- 1 small cucumber, diced
- ½ teaspoon sea salt
- 1 teaspoon dried oregano
- 1 cup full-fat grass-fed sour cream
- ½ cup full-fat Greek yogurt
- 1½ tablespoons freshly squeezed lemon juice
- 2 tablespoons fresh dill
- 1 teaspoon ground cumin
- 1 teaspoon paprika
- 1 garlic clove, minced
- ¼ teaspoon freshly ground black pepper

PREP
5 minutes

SAUTÉ
2 minutes

PRESSURE COOK
25 minutes on High

RELEASE
Natural for 10 minutes, then Quick

TOTAL
52 minutes

- GLUTEN-FREE
- NUT-FREE

PER SERVING (2 LETTUCE WRAPS)
Calories: 432; Total fat: 27g; Total carbs: 11g; Net carbs: 10g; Fiber: 1g; Sugar: 3g; Protein: 36g

MACROS
56% fat
10% carbs
34% protein

1. In a medium bowl, add 2 tablespoons of ghee and mix in the garlic, marjoram, rosemary, salt, and pepper. Add the pork to the bowl and rub with the ghee mixture. Set aside.
2. Select the pressure cooker's Sauté or Browning feature, adjust the heat to medium, and melt the remaining 2 tablespoons of ghee until shimmering. Add the sliced onion and sauté for 1 to 2 minutes. Add the seasoned pork to the pressure cooker. Pour the lemon juice and bone broth over the meat and stir.
3. Lock the lid into place and set the steam release knob to the sealed position. Set the pressure level to High and the time to 25 minutes.
4. While the pork cooks, make the tzatziki. In a small bowl, combine and mix all of the tzatziki ingredients. Set aside.
5. After the pork is finished cooking, let the pressure release naturally for 10 minutes, then quick release any remaining pressure. Unlock and remove the lid. Remove the meat and onions with a slotted spoon.
6. Serve as lettuce wraps, topped with the tzatziki, olives, and feta cheese.

MACRO TIP: Already hit your fat macros for the day? Substitute full-fat Greek yogurt for the sour cream to change the macronutrient profile of the meal so it's higher in protein and lower in fat.

Crispy Pork Carnitas

This recipe combines two of my favorites flavors, citrus and garlic. These crispy pork carnitas are tender and juicy, and done in just over one hour. My favorite pairing is carnitas served over a bed of greens with a hefty serving of delicious Guacamole (page 27). **SERVES 8**

1 tablespoon ground cumin

1 teaspoon dried oregano

1 teaspoon chili powder

1 teaspoon sea salt

½ teaspoon freshly ground black pepper

3½ pounds boneless pork roast, excess fat trimmed, cut into chunks

½ cup freshly squeezed orange juice

¼ cup freshly squeezed lime juice

¾ cup chicken broth

1 cup thinly sliced onion

6 garlic cloves, minced

1 bay leaf

4 tablespoons Ghee (page 18), divided

¼ cup chopped fresh cilantro

4 cups mixed greens

4 cups Guacamole (page 27)

PREP
15 minutes

PRESSURE COOK
30 minutes on High

RELEASE
Natural

TOTAL
1 hour 10 minutes

- GLUTEN-FREE
- NUT-FREE

PER SERVING
Calories: 559; Total fat: 34g; Total carbs: 17g; Net carbs: 8g; Fiber: 9g; Sugar: 2g; Protein: 46g

MACROS
55% fat
12% carbs
33% protein

1. In a small bowl, combine the cumin, oregano, chili powder, sea salt, and pepper. Put the pork chunks in a large bowl, sprinkle with the seasoning mixture, and toss to coat.
2. Pour the orange juice, lime juice, and chicken broth into the pressure cooker. Add the onion, garlic, and bay leaf and stir to combine. Add the spice-coated pork.

3. Lock the lid into place and set the steam release knob to the sealed position. Set the pressure level to High and the time to 30 minutes. After cooking, let the pressure release naturally. Unlock and remove the lid. Using a slotted spoon, transfer the pork to a medium bowl. Do not discard the leftover liquid from the pressure cooker. Using two forks, shred the pork meat.
4. Heat 2 tablespoons of ghee in a large skillet over high heat. Add the shredded pork to the pan in small batches and sear until the pork starts to crisp. Pour ½ cup of the leftover liquid from the pressure cooker over the pork and continue to sear until the liquid evaporates. Transfer to a platter. Repeat until all the pork has been seared, using the remaining ghee as necessary.
5. Finish by pouring some more of the remaining cooking liquid onto the seared pork and topping with the chopped cilantro.
6. Serve the carnitas over mixed greens and top with the guacamole.

COOKING TIP: Make this dish one-pot by using the Sauté or Browning feature on your pressure cooker instead of using the stove top. After you shred the pork, transfer the cooking liquid to another bowl and set the pressure cooker to Sauté or Browning. Heat 1 to 2 tablespoons of ghee in the cooker until shimmering, then add the shredded pork. Sauté with 1 cup of leftover liquid until the meat starts to crisp and the liquid evaporates.

Barbecue Pulled Pork

This pulled pork is made from pork shoulder and comes out amazingly tender and full of flavor. It cooks in my favorite Sugar-Free Barbecue Sauce *(page 26)* *and pairs perfectly with any of the Cauliflower Rice Three Ways variations* *(see page 30)*. **SERVES 8**

- 1 tablespoon garlic powder
- 1 tablespoon mustard powder
- 2 teaspoons chili powder
- 2 teaspoons sea salt
- 1 teaspoon freshly ground black pepper
- 1 teaspoon smoked paprika
- 1 teaspoon ground cumin
- 1 teaspoon ground cinnamon
- 4 pounds pork shoulder, cut into 4 (1-pound) pieces
- 2 tablespoons Ghee (page 18)
- 1 cup Sugar-Free Barbecue Sauce (page 26), plus more for serving

PREP
5 minutes

SAUTÉ
25 minutes

PRESSURE COOK
60 minutes on High

RELEASE
Natural

TOTAL
1 hour 45 minutes

- GLUTEN-FREE
- NUT-FREE

PER SERVING
Calories: 414; Total fat: 28g; Total carbs: 7g; Net carbs: 6g; Fiber: 1g; Sugar: 5g; Protein: 37g

MACROS
59% fat
7% carbs
34% protein

1. In a small bowl, combine the garlic powder, mustard powder, chili powder, salt, pepper, paprika, cumin, and cinnamon and mix well. Put the pork in a medium bowl and rub the spice mixture evenly over the pieces.
2. Select the pressure cooker's Sauté or Browning feature, adjust the heat to medium, and heat the ghee until shimmering. Working in two batches, place the pork pieces in a single layer in the pressure cooker. Cook the pork, turning frequently, for about 5 minutes per batch, or until lightly browned. As the pork finishes browning, transfer to a plate.
3. Put all the pork back in the pressure cooker and add ½ cup of water and 1 cup of barbecue sauce. Stir until well combined.

4. Lock the lid into place and set the steam release knob to the sealed position. Set the pressure level to High and the time to 60 minutes. After cooking is complete, let the pressure release naturally. Unlock and remove the lid.
5. Carefully transfer the pork to a large bowl and, using two forks, shred the meat. If the pork doesn't shred easily, return it to the pressure cooker and cook for an additional 10 to 20 minutes on High pressure, then transfer back to the bowl and shred.
6. Select the pressure cooker's Sauté or Browning feature and cook the sauce left in the cooker for 10 to 15 minutes, or until it is reduced by half. Transfer the shredded pork to the sauce and mix well. Serve with more barbecue sauce.

Hawaiian Pork

A recipe that would usually take the better part of a day to make in a smoker or slow cooker is achieved in just under two hours thanks to the convenience of the pressure cooker. This kalua pork has a melt-in-your-mouth smoky flavor and pairs perfectly with Coconut-Lime Cauliflower Rice (page 30) for that true island feel. **SERVES 8**

2 tablespoons coconut oil

4 pounds pork shoulder, cut into two pieces

6 garlic cloves, peeled

2 teaspoons pink Himalayan sea salt

1 tablespoon coconut aminos

2 teaspoons liquid smoke

1. Select the pressure cooker's Sauté or Browning feature, adjust the heat to medium, and heat the coconut oil until shimmering. Add the pork and brown on all sides, about 5 minutes. Remove the pork from the pressure cooker, transfer to a work surface, and let cool slightly.
2. Using a sharp knife, cut three slits into each piece of pork and press in the garlic cloves. Sprinkle the pink Himalayan sea salt evenly over the pork.
3. Pour ½ cup of water into the pressure cooker and add the coconut aminos, liquid smoke, and browned pork.
4. Lock the lid into place and set the steam release knob to the sealed position. Set the pressure level to High and the time to 90 minutes. After cooking, let the pressure release naturally. Unlock and remove the lid.
5. Use tongs to carefully remove the pork from the pressure cooker and transfer to a large bowl. Using two forks, shred the pork before serving.

PREP
3 minutes

SAUTÉ
5 minutes

PRESSURE COOK
90 minutes on High

RELEASE
Natural

TOTAL
1 hour 48 minutes

- DAIRY-FREE
- GLUTEN-FREE
- NUT-FREE

PER SERVING (½ POUND)
Calories: 517; Total fat: 36g; Total carbs: 1g; Net carbs: 1g; Fiber: 0g; Sugar: 1g; Protein: 44g

MACROS
64% fat
1% carbs
35% protein

Pork Belly

Do you know what's better than bacon? Pork belly! Pork belly is basically uncured, unsmoked, unsliced bacon, and it is a complete delicacy. Luckily, it can also be made in a fraction of the time using a pressure cooker. **SERVES 8**

1 tablespoon paprika

1 tablespoon dried thyme

1 tablespoon dried oregano

1 tablespoon sea salt

1 teaspoon ground cloves

½ teaspoon freshly ground black pepper

6 garlic cloves, minced

1 pound skinless pork belly

¾ cup dry white wine

2 tablespoons avocado oil

1. In a small bowl, mix together the paprika, thyme, oregano, salt, cloves, pepper, and garlic.
2. Using a sharp knife, cut diagonal lines across the fattier side of the pork going one way, then repeat going the opposite direction, to create a diamond pattern in the fat. Rub the pork fat with the spice mixture.
3. Pour the wine into the pressure cooker, then place the pork belly in the cooker spice-rubbed-side up. Lock the lid into place and set the steam release knob to the sealed position. Set the pressure level to High and the time to 30 minutes. After cooking, quick release the pressure.
4. Unlock and remove the lid. Transfer the pork belly to a cutting board and let sit for 5 to 8 minutes to cool slightly. Cut into ¼-inch-thick slices (or your desired thickness).
5. Heat the avocado oil in a large skillet over medium-high heat. Add the pork slices and sear for a minute or two on each side, or until desired crispness is reached.

PREP
8 minutes

SAUTÉ
10 minutes

PRESSURE COOK
30 minutes on High

RELEASE
Quick

TOTAL
58 minutes

- DAIRY-FREE
- GLUTEN-FREE
- NUT-FREE

PER SERVING
Calories: 355; Total fat: 34g; Total carbs: 2g; Net carbs: 1g; Fiber: 1g; Sugar: 0.5g; Protein: 6g

MACROS
90% fat
3% carbs
7% protein

Fall-off-the-Bone Baby Back Ribs

Before my Instant Pot, I would cook ribs in a slow cooker for the better part of a day. This recipe lets me make finger-licking baby back ribs in an hour, so I never have to plan too far ahead. This recipe calls for my Sugar-Free Barbecue Sauce (page 26). **SERVES 4**

- 1 tablespoon paprika
- 1 tablespoon garlic powder
- 1 tablespoon onion powder
- 2 tablespoons chili powder
- ½ teaspoon cayenne pepper
- 2 teaspoons dried oregano
- 1 rack baby back pork ribs
- ¼ cup apple cider vinegar
- ¼ teaspoon liquid smoke
- 1 cup Sugar-Free Barbecue Sauce (page 26), divided

1. In a small bowl, mix the paprika, garlic powder, onion powder, chili powder, cayenne pepper, and oregano and set aside.
2. Remove the membrane from the bottom side of the ribs by inserting the tip of a knife under the skin to get it started. Grip and remove the membrane completely. Rub the spice mixture evenly over the ribs.
3. Pour 1 cup of water into the pressure cooker and add the cider vinegar and liquid smoke. Place a trivet inside and place the ribs on top of the trivet.
4. Lock the lid into place and set the steam release knob to the sealed position. Set the pressure level to High and the time to 25 minutes. After cooking, let the pressure release naturally. Unlock and remove the lid.

PREP
8 minutes

PRESSURE COOK
25 minutes on High

BROIL
5 minutes

RELEASE
Natural

TOTAL
1 hour

- DAIRY-FREE
- GLUTEN-FREE
- NUT-FREE

PER SERVING
Calories: 511; Total fat: 31g; Total carbs: 12g; Net carbs: 8g; Fiber: 4g; Sugar: 4g; Protein: 22g

MACROS
66% fat
12% carbs
22% protein

5. Preheat the oven to broil. Line a baking sheet with parchment paper.
6. Carefully remove the ribs from the pressure cooker and place on the prepared baking sheet. Brush with ½ cup of barbecue sauce and broil for 3 to 5 minutes. Remove from the oven and serve hot with the rest of the barbecue sauce for dipping.

COOKING TIP: I love my ribs cooked so they fall off the bone, but you can adjust the cook time to your liking. Sixteen minutes will result in ribs that are tender with some chew, while 25 minutes results in fall-off-the-bone tender ribs.

Kielbasa and Sauerkraut

Sauerkraut is a love-it-or-hate-it type of food—and I love it. This recipe combines sauerkraut with savory sausage and the sweetness of carrot and apple to create a delicious dish. **SERVES 6**

- 8 bacon slices, chopped
- 4 tablespoons Ghee (page 18)
- 1 yellow onion, sliced
- 4 garlic cloves, minced
- 1 large carrot, peeled and diced
- ½ apple, peeled and grated
- 1 teaspoon dried thyme
- ½ teaspoon dried sage
- ⅓ cup dry white wine
- 1 teaspoon sea salt
- ½ teaspoon freshly ground black pepper
- 1 pound kielbasa, cut into bite-size pieces
- 1 (16-ounce) jar sauerkraut
- ½ cup Bone Broth (page 19) or chicken broth
- Chopped fresh parsley, for serving

PREP
5 minutes

SAUTÉ
10 minutes

PRESSURE COOK
5 minutes on High

RELEASE
Quick

TOTAL
30 minutes

- GLUTEN-FREE
- NUT-FREE

PER SERVING
Calories: 377; Total fat: 23g; Total carbs: 13g; Net carbs: 8g; Fiber: 5g; Sugar: 6g; Protein: 17g

MACROS
63% fat
16% carbs
21% protein

1. Select the pressure cooker's Sauté or Browning feature, adjust the heat to medium, and sauté the chopped bacon until browned. Transfer the bacon to paper towels to drain and pour off the fat from the pressure cooker.
2. Melt the ghee in the pressure cooker. Add the onion, garlic, and carrot and sauté until the carrot has softened. Add the apple, thyme, sage, wine, salt, and pepper and cook for 1 to 2 minutes, or until the liquid is reduced by about half.

3. Add the cooked bacon, kielbasa, sauerkraut, and broth to the pressure cooker. Mix well to combine the ingredients and ensure that nothing is stuck to the bottom of the pan.
4. Lock the lid into place and set the steam release knob to the sealed position. Set the pressure level to High and the time to 5 minutes. After cooking, quick release the pressure. Unlock and remove the lid. Serve the kielbasa and sauerkraut topped with chopped parsley.

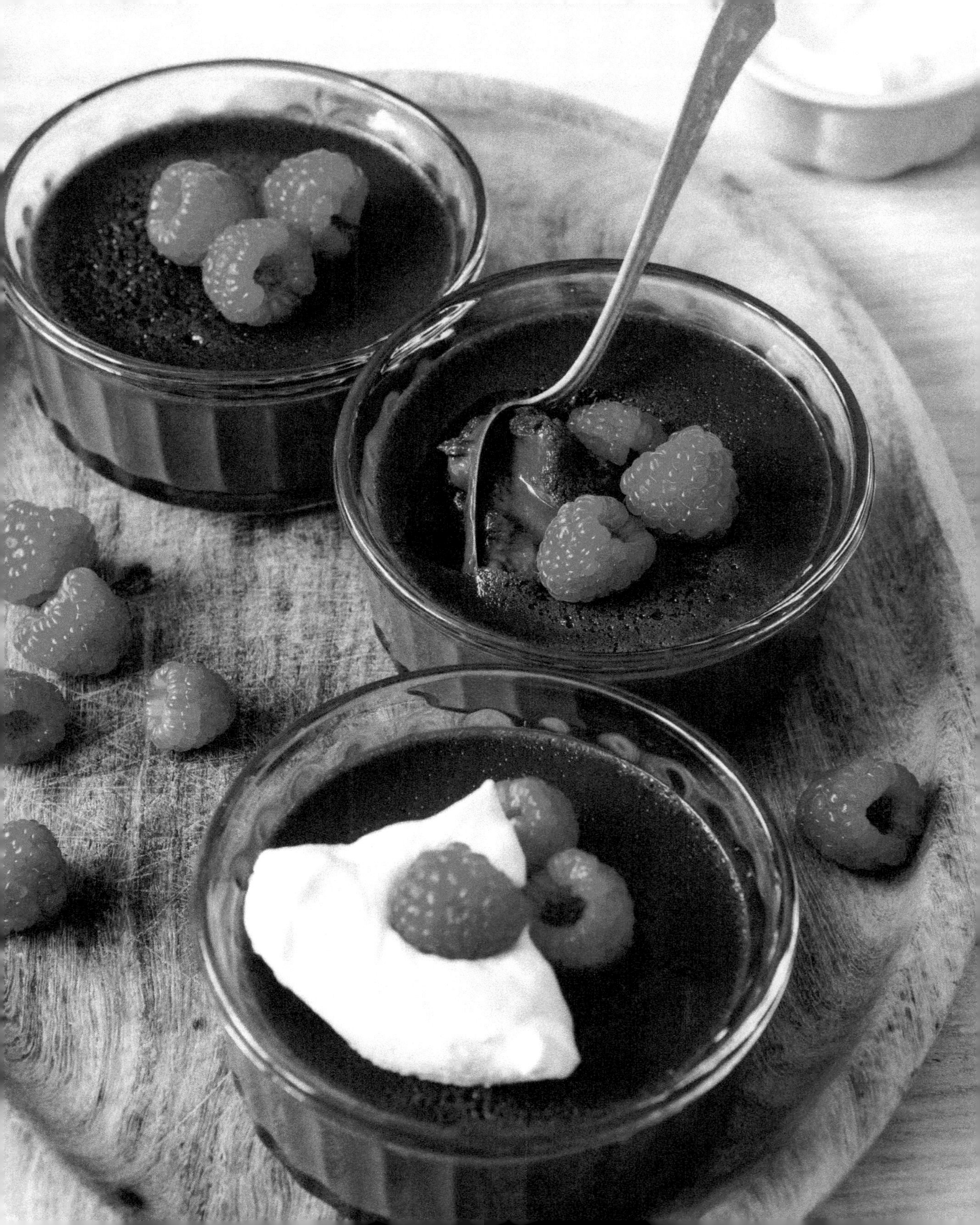

Chapter Nine

Desserts

(left) Chocolate Mousse

Key Lime Pie

Sweetened condensed milk is an ingredient in one of my favorite desserts, Key lime pie. Discovering how to make Sugar-Free Sweetened Condensed Milk (page 20) means that it is now possible for me to make this pie keto-friendly. Though I avoid eating desserts on a regular basis, when the right occasion calls for it, this Key lime pie is one of my go-to options. **SERVES 6**

FOR THE CRUST

4 tablespoons unsalted grass-fed butter, melted, plus more for greasing

1 cup almond flour

6 to 8 teaspoons liquid stevia or preferred powdered sugar substitute equivalent to 1 tablespoon sugar

FOR THE FILLING

4 large egg yolks

1⅓ cups Sugar-Free Sweetened Condensed Milk (page 20)

½ cup freshly squeezed Key lime juice

½ cup full-fat sour cream

3 tablespoons finely grated Key lime zest

FOR THE TOPPING

1 cup heavy cream

6 to 8 teaspoons liquid stevia or preferred powdered sugar substitute equivalent to 1 tablespoon sugar

1 teaspoon vanilla extract

1 tablespoon finely grated Key lime zest, for garnish (optional)

PREP
20 minutes

PRESSURE COOK
15 minutes on High

RELEASE
Natural for 10 minutes, then Quick

TOTAL
55 minutes, plus at least 4 hours to chill

- GLUTEN-FREE
- VEGETARIAN

PER SERVING
Calories: 270; Total fat: 25g; Total carbs: 8g; Net carbs: 7g; Fiber: 1g; Sugar: 3g; Protein: 4g

MACROS
83% fat
12% carbs
5% protein

To make the crust

1. Grease a 7-inch springform pan with butter.
2. In a small bowl, mix the almond flour, 4 tablespoons of butter, and the stevia.
3. Press the mixture evenly into the bottom and up the side of the springform pan. Freeze the piecrust for 15 minutes.

To make the filling

1. In a medium bowl, using a handheld electric mixer, beat the egg yolks for 2 to 3 minutes, or until pale yellow and starting to thicken. While continuing to mix, gradually add the condensed milk, lime juice, sour cream, and lime zest. Continue to mix until smooth. Pour the pie filling into the crust in the springform pan and cover with aluminum foil.
2. Pour 1 cup of water into the pressure cooker and place the trivet inside.
3. Make a sling with aluminum foil by folding a long piece of foil into thirds. Use the sling to lower the springform pan into the pressure cooker.
4. Lock the lid into place and set the steam release knob to the sealed position. Set the pressure level to High and the time to 15 minutes. After cooking, let the pressure release naturally for 10 minutes, then quick release any remaining pressure. Unlock and remove the lid.
5. Using the foil sling, carefully remove the pie from the pressure cooker. Let cool at room temperature for 10 to 15 minutes, then transfer to the refrigerator to chill for at least 4 hours or overnight, until ready to serve.

To make the topping

About 20 minutes before serving, place a metal mixing bowl in the freezer for 15 minutes. Remove the bowl and add the cream, stevia, and vanilla, and beat with the handheld electric mixer until medium peaks form, about 1 to 2 minutes. Serve the pie immediately with the whipped cream, garnished with the lime zest (if using).

Cheesecake

My favorite thing about this recipe is the texture. The creamy, smooth filling is balanced out perfectly by the crunch of the nut-and-coconut-filled crust. You can easily switch out the macadamia nuts for the nut of your choice for a different variation. **SERVES 6**

FOR THE CRUST

3 tablespoons unsalted grass-fed butter, plus more for greasing

1 cup macadamia nuts

⅓ cup almond flour

⅓ cup shredded coconut

6 to 9 drops liquid stevia or preferred powdered sugar substitute equivalent to 1 tablespoon sugar

½ teaspoon sea salt

FOR THE FILLING

16 ounces cream cheese, at room temperature

½ cup organic sour cream

1 tablespoon freshly squeezed lemon juice

Finely grated zest of 1 lemon

1 tablespoon vanilla extract

¼ teaspoon liquid stevia or ¼ cup preferred powdered sugar substitute

2 large eggs, at room temperature

FOR THE TOPPING

½ cup sour cream

1 teaspoon preferred powdered sugar substitute

PREP
15 minutes

PRESSURE COOK
35 minutes on High

RELEASE
Natural

TOTAL
1 hour 10 minutes, plus 6 to 8 hours to chill

- GLUTEN-FREE
- VEGETARIAN

PER SERVING
Calories: 594; Total fat: 25g; Total carbs: 16g; Net carbs: 11g; Fiber: 5g; Sugar: 5g; Protein: 11g

MACROS
82% fat
10% carbs
8% protein

To make the crust

1. Preheat the oven to 350°F. Grease a 7-inch springform pan with butter.
2. In a food processor, pulse the macadamia nuts until they are crushed. In a small bowl, mix the crushed macadamias with the almond flour, shredded coconut, 3 tablespoons of butter, the stevia, and salt. Press the mixture evenly into the bottom and up the side of the springform pan.
3. Bake the crust for 8 minutes. Promptly remove from the oven and let cool.

To make the filling

1. While the crust is baking, prepare the filling. In a medium bowl, combine the cream cheese, sour cream, lemon juice, lemon zest, vanilla extract, and stevia. Using a handheld electric mixer, blend until smooth. Add one egg at a time and gently mix until just combined. Do not overmix or the cheesecake will lose the desired creamy texture. Pour the cheesecake filling into the crust in the springform pan and cover with aluminum foil.
2. Pour 1 cup of water into the pressure cooker and place the trivet inside.
3. Make a sling with aluminum foil by folding a long piece of foil into thirds. Use the sling to lower the springform pan onto the trivet in the pressure cooker.
4. Lock the lid into place and set the steam release knob to the sealed position. Set the pressure level to High and the time to 35 minutes.
5. After cooking is complete, let the pressure release naturally. Unlock and remove the lid.
6. Using the foil sling, carefully remove the cheesecake from the pressure cooker and gently dab any moisture off the top of the cake with a paper towel.

To make the topping

1. While the cheesecake is cooking, in a small bowl, mix the sour cream and sugar substitute. Set aside.
2. While the cheesecake is still hot, evenly spread the topping over it.
3. Refrigerate the cheesecake for 6 to 8 hours before serving.

PREP TIP: Short on time? Make this a crustless cheesecake by lining the springform pan with parchment paper. This drops the calories to 381 per serving, and the total carbs to 9 grams per serving.

Crème Brûlée

Crème brûlée is a rich custard topped with a hard caramel crust. Enjoy with some raspberries, and this high-fat dessert is sure to impress. **SERVES 6**

- Unsalted grass-fed butter, for greasing
- 6 large egg yolks
- ½ teaspoon liquid stevia or preferred powdered sugar substitute equivalent to ½ cup sugar
- ⅛ teaspoon sea salt
- 2 cups heavy cream
- 1 teaspoon vanilla extract
- 6 tablespoons powdered sugar substitute, for topping (use one with a 1:1 substitution ratio to sugar)
- ½ cup fresh raspberries

1. Lightly grease six ramekins with butter.
2. In a medium bowl, whisk together the egg yolks, stevia, and salt. Add the cream and vanilla extract and mix until smooth. Pour the mixture into the prepared ramekins. Cover each with aluminum foil.
3. Pour 1 cup of water into the pressure cooker and place the trivet inside. Place three of the ramekins on the trivet. Stack the remaining three ramekins on top of the first three ramekins.
4. Lock the lid into place and set the steam release knob to the sealed position. Set the pressure level to High and the time to 6 minutes. After cooking, let the pressure release naturally for 10 minutes, then quick release any remaining pressure. Unlock and remove the lid.

PREP
5 minutes

PRESSURE COOK
6 minutes on High

RELEASE
Natural for 10 minutes, then Quick

BROIL
10 minutes

TOTAL
40 minutes, plus 2 to 4 hours to chill

- GLUTEN-FREE
- NUT-FREE
- VEGETARIAN

PER SERVING
Calories: 336; Total fat: 34g; Total carbs: 4g; Net carbs: 3g; Fiber: 1g; Sugar: 3g; Protein: 4g

MACROS
91% fat
3% carbs
6% protein

5. Carefully remove the ramekins from the pressure cooker and discard the foil. Allow to cool. Cover with plastic wrap and refrigerate for 2 to 4 hours.
6. Before serving, remove the ramekins from the refrigerator and top each with 1 tablespoon of powdered sugar substitute. Using a kitchen torch, move the flame 2 inches above the surface of each custard until it forms a hard, caramelized crust. Let cool and serve topped with the raspberries.

INGREDIENT SUBSTITUTION: Make this dessert dairy-free by using coconut oil instead of butter to grease the ramekins and substituting coconut cream for the heavy cream.

Chocolate Mousse

Craving chocolate? This dense, creamy chocolate mousse made with stevia-sweetened chocolate is the answer to all the keto chocolate-lover's dreams. This recipe can be made with individual glass ramekins or a springform pan, but the cooking time will be different depending on which you use. The main method and associated times apply if you are using ramekins. See the Cooking Tip to use a springform pan. Serve this recipe with whipped cream and raspberries to create the perfect flavor combination. **SERVES 4**

- 1½ cups heavy cream
- ½ cup whole milk
- 6 ounces Lily's stevia-sweetened chocolate chips or chopped sugar-free chocolate
- 5 large eggs yolks
- ¼ teaspoon liquid stevia or ¼ cup preferred powdered sugar substitute
- 2 teaspoons vanilla extract
- ¼ teaspoon pink Himalayan sea salt
- 1 cup whipped cream, for serving
- ½ cup fresh raspberries

PREP
5 minutes

PRESSURE COOK
10 minutes on High

RELEASE
Natural for 5 minutes, then Quick

TOTAL
25 minutes, plus at least 3 hours to chill

- GLUTEN-FREE
- NUT-FREE
- VEGETARIAN

PER SERVING
Calories: 421; Total fat: 37g; Total carbs: 17g; Net carbs: 9g; Fiber: 8g; Sugar: 3g; Protein: 7g

MACROS
77% fat
16% carbs
7% protein

1. In a medium saucepan, bring the cream and milk to a simmer over medium heat. Once simmering, remove the pot from the heat and add the chocolate. Whisk until melted and smooth.
2. In a large bowl, whisk together the egg yolks, stevia, vanilla, and pink Himalayan sea salt. While stirring, pour the chocolate mixture into the yolk mixture in a thin stream, stirring constantly.

3. Pour the chocolate and yolk mixture into 4 or 5 heat-proof dessert glasses or ramekins. If all 5 glasses do not fit, you will need to pressure cook the remaining ones separately, but there is no change to the cooking time. This recipe can be made with individual glass ramekins or a springform pan, but the cooking time will be different depending on which you use. The main method and associated times apply if you are using ramekins. See the Cooking Tip to use a springform pan.
4. Pour 2 cups of water into the pressure cooker and place the trivet inside. Arrange the glasses on the trivet.
5. Lock the lid into place and set the steam release knob to the sealed position. Set the pressure level to High and the time to 10 minutes. After cooking is complete, let the pressure release naturally for 5 minutes, then quick release any remaining pressure. Unlock and remove the lid.
6. Let the glasses cool in the pressure cooker pot for 5 to 8 minutes before removing them. Refrigerate for at least 3 hours or overnight. Serve with the whipped cream and raspberries.

COOKING TIP:
Instead of cooking the mousse in individual glasses, you can also make it in a 7-inch springform pan. To do so, pour the chocolate and yolk mixture into the pan in step 3. Cover loosely with aluminum foil. Pour 1 cup of water into the pressure cooker and place the trivet inside. Make a sling with aluminum foil by folding a long piece of foil lengthwise into thirds. Use the sling to lower the pan of mousse onto the trivet in the pressure cooker. Increase the pressure cooking time to 18 minutes, and follow the instructions as written for pressure release.

Lemon Custard

This recipe results in the most refreshing and light citrus flavors. Topped with fresh raspberries, blackberries, and strawberries, this custard is the perfect spring or summer dessert. **SERVES 4**

1 cup full-fat coconut cream

3 tablespoons unsalted grass-fed butter, at room temperature

4 large egg yolks plus 1 large egg

½ teaspoon liquid stevia or ½ cup preferred powdered sugar substitute

1 teaspoon vanilla extract

3 tablespoons freshly squeezed lemon juice

2 teaspoons finely grated lemon zest

1 cup mixed fresh berries

1. In a food processor or blender, mix the coconut cream, butter, egg yolks, whole egg, stevia, vanilla, lemon juice, and lemon zest until smooth.
2. Pour the mixture into a 7-inch round pan that fits into the pressure cooker. Cover tightly with foil.
3. Pour 1 cup of water into the pressure cooker and place the trivet inside. Make a sling with aluminum foil by folding a long piece of foil lengthwise into thirds. Use the sling to lower the custard pan onto the trivet in the pressure cooker.

PREP
5 minutes

PRESSURE COOK
10 minutes on High

RELEASE
Quick

TOTAL
25 minutes, plus 2 hours to chill

- GLUTEN-FREE
- NUT-FREE
- VEGETARIAN

PER SERVING
Calories: 267; Total fat: 24g; Total carbs: 9g; Net carbs: 7g; Fiber: 2g; Sugar: 5g; Protein: 6g

MACROS
78% fat
13% carbs
9% protein

4. Lock the lid into place and set the steam release knob to the sealed position. Set the pressure level to High and the time to 10 minutes. After cooking, quick release the pressure. Unlock and remove the lid.
5. Using the foil sling, carefully remove the custard pan from the pressure cooker. Remove and discard the foil and place the custard in the refrigerator for 1 to 2 hours to chill before servings with the fresh berries.

Marbled Pumpkin Cheesecake

What do you get when you cross pumpkin pie and cheesecake? This delicious dessert! A pecan crust provides just the right amount of crunch for the smooth filling. It's perfect for Thanksgiving, or any time of year. **SERVES 8**

FOR THE CRUST

1 cup finely chopped pecans, toasted

1 tablespoon Swerve granulated sweetener

2 tablespoons unsalted grass-fed butter, softened

FOR THE FILLING

8 ounces cream cheese, softened

6 tablespoons full-fat sour cream, at room temperature

½ cup Swerve granulated sweetener

2 large eggs

1 cup pumpkin purée

1¼ teaspoon pumpkin pie spice

PREP
10 minutes

PRESSURE COOK
30 minutes on High

RELEASE
Natural for 10 minutes, then Quick

TOTAL
1 hour, plus 4 to 5 hours to chill

- GLUTEN-FREE
- VEGETARIAN

PER SERVING
Calories: 272; Total fat: 26g; Total carbs: 6g; Net carbs: 4g; Fiber: 2g; Sugar: 3g; Protein: 5g

MACROS
83% fat
9% carbs
8% protein

To make the crust

1. In a food processor, process the pecans and Swerve until the nuts are very finely chopped. Add the butter and process until a coarse paste forms.
2. Press the mixture into the bottom of a 7-inch spring-form pan and up the side about ½ inch. Chill the crust in the refrigerator while you make the filling.

To make the filling

In a medium bowl, using a handheld electric mixer, beat the cream cheese and sour cream until very smooth. Add the Swerve and beat until smooth. Add the eggs and beat just to blend. Remove about ⅓ cup of the cream cheese mixture and set aside. Add the pumpkin purée and pumpkin pie spice to the mixture in the bowl and beat until well blended.

1. Pour the pumpkin mixture over the crust in the springform pan. Place 5 or 6 spoonfuls of the reserved cream cheese mixture evenly over the top of the pumpkin mixture and drag the tip of a knife or a skewer through the cream cheese dollops to make a marbleized pattern on the top.
2. Pour 1 cup of water into the pressure cooker and place a trivet with handles inside. Place the springform pan on top of the trivet. Make a sling with aluminum foil by folding a long piece of foil into thirds. Use the sling to lower the pan onto the trivet in the pressure cooker. Lock the lid into place and set the steam release knob to the sealed position. Set the pressure level to High and the time to 30 minutes. After cooking, let the pressure release naturally for 10 minutes, then quick release any remaining pressure. Unlock and remove the lid.
3. Carefully remove the cheesecake from the pressure cooker and remove the foil. The cheesecake should be set; use a skewer to test the center. If it's not quite done, return it to the cooker, close and lock the lid, and let sit, not under pressure, for another few minutes.
4. Let the cheesecake cool for 15 to 20 minutes at room temperature, then refrigerate for 4 to 5 hours to set completely before serving.

Mini Coconut-Ricotta Custard Cups

These rich custard desserts are a delightful twist on the typical ricotta cheesecake. A hint of coconut milk and toasted coconut gives them an intriguing flavor that's sure to please any coconut lover. **SERVES 6**

8 ounces cream cheese, softened

⅔ cup full-fat ricotta cheese

½ cup coconut milk

⅔ cup Swerve granulated sweetener

1 teaspoon vanilla extract

2 large eggs plus 2 large egg yolks

½ cup toasted unsweetened shredded coconut

PREP
10 minutes

PRESSURE COOK
6 minutes on High

RELEASE
Natural for 10 minutes, then Quick

TOTAL
35 minutes, plus 2 to 4 hours to chill

- GLUTEN-FREE
- NUT-FREE
- VEGETARIAN

PER SERVING
Calories: 276; Total fat: 2g; Total carbs: 5g; Net carbs: 5g; Fiber: 1g; Sugar: 3g; Protein: 9g

MACROS
80% fat
7% carbs
13% protein

1. In a medium bowl, using a handheld electric mixer, beat the cream cheese, ricotta, and coconut milk until very smooth. Add the Swerve and vanilla and beat until smooth. Add the whole eggs and egg yolks and beat just to blend. Stir in the shredded coconut.
2. Pour the custard mixture evenly into six 1- to 1½-cup ramekins, leaving about ½ inch of space at the top of each ramekin. Cover the ramekins with aluminum foil.
3. Pour 1 cup of water into the pressure cooker and place the trivet inside. Place three of the ramekins on the trivet. Stack the remaining three ramekins on top of them, staggering them slightly.

4. Lock the lid into place and set the steam release knob to the sealed position. Set the pressure level to High and the time to 6 minutes. After cooking, let the pressure release naturally for 10 minutes, then quick release any remaining pressure. Unlock and remove the lid.
5. Carefully remove the foil from one of the ramekins and check to see if the custard is done. If it's not quite set in the center, lock the pressure cooker lid back into place and cook on High for another 5 minutes or so. Carefully remove the ramekins and discard the foil. Let the custards cool. Cover with plastic wrap and refrigerate for 2 to 4 hours before serving.

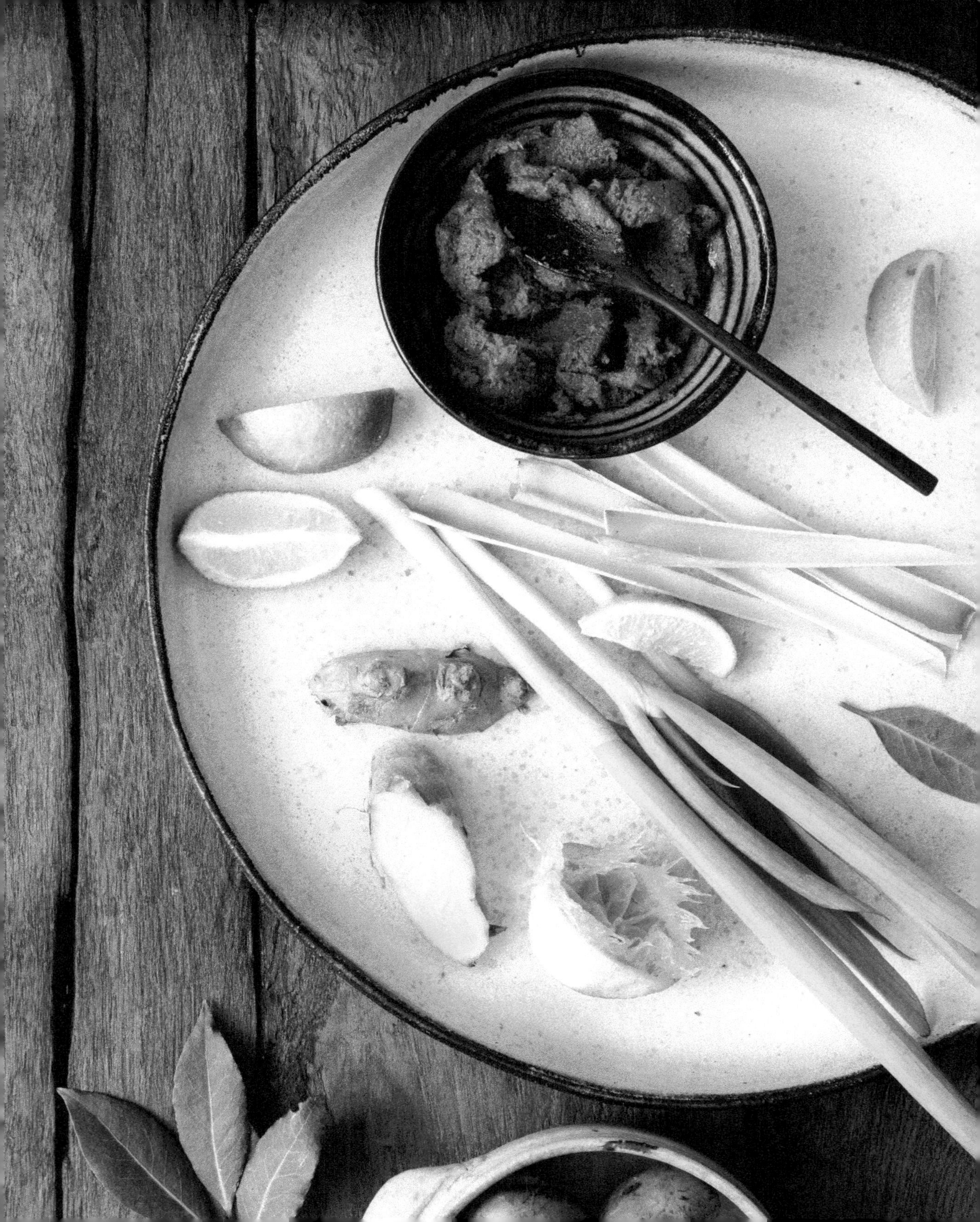

PRESSURE COOKING TIME CHARTS

The following charts provide approximate cooking times for a variety of foods. To begin, you may want to cook for a minute or two less than the times listed; you can always simmer foods at natural pressure to finish cooking.

Keep in mind that these times are for the foods partially submerged in water (or broth) or steamed, and for the foods cooked alone. The cooking times for the same foods when they are part of a recipe may differ because of additional ingredients or cooking liquids, or a different release method than the one listed here.

For any foods labeled with "Natural" release, allow at least 15 minutes natural pressure release before quick releasing any remaining pressure.

MEAT

Except as noted, these times are for braised meats—that is, meats that are seared before pressure cooking and partially submerged in liquid.

MEAT	MINUTES UNDER PRESSURE	PRESSURE	RELEASE
BEEF, SHOULDER (CHUCK) ROAST (2 LB.)	35	High	Natural
BEEF, SHOULDER (CHUCK), 2" CHUNKS	20	High	Natural for 10 minutes
BEEF, BONE-IN SHORT RIBS	40	High	Natural
BEEF, FLAT IRON STEAK, CUT INTO ½" STRIPS	1	Low	Quick
BEEF, SIRLOIN STEAK, CUT INTO ½" STRIPS	1	Low	Quick
LAMB, SHOULDER, 2" CHUNKS	35	High	Natural
LAMB, SHANKS	40	High	Natural
PORK, SHOULDER ROAST (2 LB.)	25	High	Natural

MEAT	MINUTES UNDER PRESSURE	PRESSURE	RELEASE
PORK, SHOULDER, 2" CHUNKS	20	High	Natural
PORK, TENDERLOIN	4	Low	Quick
PORK, BACK RIBS (STEAMED)	30	High	Quick
PORK, SPARE RIBS (STEAMED)	20	High	Quick
PORK, SMOKED SAUSAGE, ½" SLICES	20	High	Quick

FISH AND SEAFOOD

All times are for steamed fish and shellfish.

FISH AND SEAFOOD	MINUTES UNDER PRESSURE	PRESSURE	RELEASE
CLAMS	2	High	Quick
MUSSELS	1	High	Quick
SALMON, FRESH (1" THICK)	5	Low	Quick
HALIBUT, FRESH (1" THICK)	3	High	Quick
TILAPIA OR COD, FRESH	1	Low	Quick
TILAPIA OR COD, FROZEN	3	Low	Quick
LARGE SHRIMP, FROZEN	1	Low	Quick

POULTRY

Except as noted, these times are for braised poultry—that is, partially submerged in liquid.

POULTRY	MINUTES UNDER PRESSURE	PRESSURE	RELEASE
CHICKEN BREAST, BONE-IN (STEAMED)	8	Low	Natural for 5 minutes
CHICKEN BREAST, BONELESS (STEAMED)	5	Low	Natural for 8 minutes
CHICKEN THIGH, BONE-IN	15	High	Natural for 10 minutes
CHICKEN THIGH, BONELESS	8	High	Natural for 10 minutes
CHICKEN THIGH, BONELESS, 1"–2" PIECES	5	High	Quick
CHICKEN, WHOLE (SEARED ON ALL SIDES)	12–14	Low	Natural for 8 minutes
DUCK QUARTERS, BONE-IN	35	High	Quick
TURKEY BREAST, TENDERLOIN (12 OZ.) (STEAMED)	5	Low	Natural for 8 minutes
TURKEY THIGH, BONE-IN	30	High	Natural

VEGETABLES

The cooking method for all the following vegetables is steaming; if the vegetables are cooked in liquid, the times may vary. Green vegetables will be tender-crisp; root vegetables will be soft.

VEGETABLES	PREP	MINUTES UNDER PRESSURE	PRESSURE	RELEASE
ARTICHOKES, LARGE	Whole	15	High	Quick
BROCCOLI	Cut into florets	1	Low	Quick
BRUSSELS SPROUTS	Halved	2	High	Quick
CABBAGE	Sliced	5	High	Quick
CAULIFLOWER	Whole	6	High	Quick
CAULIFLOWER	Cut into florets	1	Low	Quick
GREEN BEANS	Cut in half or thirds	1	Low	Quick
SPAGHETTI SQUASH	Halved lengthwise	7	High	Quick

RESOURCES AND BRAND RECOMMENDATIONS

There is no one-size-fits-all approach to nutrition. I highly encourage you to do your research and discover what works best for you. I've listed here some of the resources that have been most helpful to me. Beyond knowledge, the quality of food you eat is as important as what you eat. On the next page is a selection of brands that make high-quality keto-compliant foods, as well as a link to my website with discount codes to help you save money.

BOOKS

The Art and Science of Low Carbohydrate Living by Jeff S. Volek, PhD, RD, and Stephen D. Phinney, MD, PhD
The Keto Diet Reset by Mark Sisson
The Big Fat Surprise by Nina Teicholz
The Ketogenic Bible by Jacob Wilson, Ph.D., and Ryan P. Lowery
Keto Clarity and *The Keto Cure* by Jimmy Moore
The Keto Diet by Leanne Vogel
Keto by Maria Emmerich and Craig Emmerich

PODCASTS

The Keto Answers Podcast with Anthony Gustin
The Keto Diet Podcast with Leanne Vogel
The Obesity Code Podcast with Dr. Jason Fung and Megan Ramos
The Primal Blueprint Podcast with Mark Sisson
The Ketogenic Athlete Podcast with Brian Williamson and Danny Vega
Ben Greenfield Fitness

WEBSITES

HealthfulPursuit.com
DietDoctor.com
PrimalBlueprint.com
Ruled.me
FitKetoGirls.com

FAVORITE BRANDS

Check out https://linktr.ee/janehdownes to find discount codes for the following brands, as well as more of my favorites!

Primal Kitchen
https://www.primalkitchen.com

Pederson Farms
http://pedersonsfarms.com

Butcher Box
https://www.butcherbox.com

Kasandrinos Olive Oil
https://kasandrinos.com

Vital Proteins
https://www.vitalproteins.com

Vital Farms Eggs
https://vitalfarms.com

Perfect Keto
https://www.perfectketo.com

MEASUREMENT CONVERSIONS

VOLUME EQUIVALENTS (LIQUID)

STANDARD	US STANDARD (OUNCES)	METRIC (APPROXIMATE)
2 tablespoons	1 fl. oz.	30 mL
¼ cup	2 fl. oz.	60 mL
½ cup	4 fl. oz.	120 mL
1 cup	8 fl. oz.	240 mL
1½ cups	12 fl. oz.	355 mL
2 cups or 1 pint	16 fl. oz.	475 mL
4 cups or 1 quart	32 fl. oz.	1 L
1 gallon	128 fl. oz.	4 L

VOLUME EQUIVALENTS (DRY)

STANDARD	METRIC (APPROXIMATE)
teaspoon	0.5 mL
¼ teaspoon	1 mL
½ teaspoon	2 mL
¾ teaspoon	4 mL
1 teaspoon	5 mL
1 tablespoon	15 mL
¼ cup	59 mL
cup	79 mL
½ cup	118 mL
cup	156 mL
¾ cup	177 mL
1 cup	235 mL
2 cups or 1 pint	475 mL
3 cups	700 mL
4 cups or 1 quart	1 L

OVEN TEMPERATURES

FAHRENHEIT (F)	CELSIUS (C) (APPROXIMATE)
250°F	120°C
300°F	150°C
325°F	165°C
350°F	180°C
375°F	190°C
400°F	200°C
425°F	220°C
450°F	230°C

WEIGHT EQUIVALENTS

STANDARD	METRIC (APPROXIMATE)
½ ounce	15 g
1 ounce	30 g
2 ounces	60 g
4 ounces	115 g
8 ounces	225 g
12 ounces	340 g
16 ounces or 1 pound	455 g

RECIPE INDEX

INDEX

W

X

Z

ACKNOWLEDGMENTS

I am extremely grateful for the amount of support I received throughout this process. I could not have done it without the love and encouragement of my friends and family.

I want to thank my parents and brother for everything they have done to support me in finding my way and pursuing my passion, for testing and retesting recipes with ingredients unavailable in Costa Rica, and for loving me, in all my forms.

To Diana, Megan, and Brandy, for helping me perfect my recipes and for believing in me. To Stacy, Janet, and everyone at Callisto Media for your expertise and help through the writing process and all that went into creating this book.

To my business partner and dear friend, Liz Williams, for the endless support both with the book and life. You paved the way, and I would not want to be on this crazy journey with anyone else.

To Suus and Dennis, for taste-tasting and critiquing my recipes, as well as for putting up with the endless dishes in the kitchen.

Thank you to my FitKetoGirls community, my Instagram followers, and everyone who has supported my journey. Your stories, experiences, and health and lifestyle transformations motivate me to continue to share my story. You inspire me every day. I would not be able to do any of this without all of you!

And, lastly, to the reader, I hope this book brings you the same health and wellness that I have found implementing this lifestyle.

XOXO

Jane

ABOUT THE AUTHOR

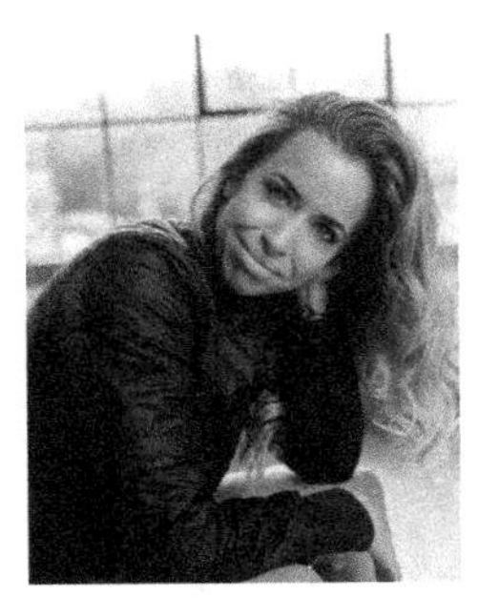

Jane Downes has worked as a personal trainer and nutrition coach since 2013. She has serviced more than 5,000 one-on-one training sessions and helped hundreds more clients through her online training and nutrition programs. She discovered the keto diet while looking for relief from anxiety and depression through a non-medication approach. She not only found the relief she was looking for but also saw amazing results in her body composition, sustainable energy, better sleep quality, improved digestion, healthier skin, and many other health benefits. Jane now specializes in helping clients create a low-carb or ketogenic lifestyle to achieve similar results. Wanting to share her results and help even more people, she co-founded the popular blog FitKetoGirls. She also shares her journey and experiences on her popular Instagram account, @janehdownes. Jane currently resides in Costa Rica.

CPSIA information can be obtained
at www.ICGtesting.com
Printed in the USA
BVHW06s1102140818
524375BV00001B/1/P

9 781939 754400